Living Allergy Free

Living Allergy Free

*How to Create and Maintain
an Allergen- and Irritant-Free
Environment*

by

M. Eric Gershwin, MD

and

Edwin L. Klingelhofer, PhD

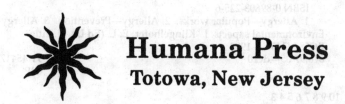

Humana Press
Totowa, New Jersey

Printed in the United States of America.

Library of Congress Cataloging in Publication Data

Main entry under title:

Gershwin, M. Eric, 1946–
     Living Allergy Free: how to create and maintain an allergen- and irritant-free environment/ by M. Eric Gershwin and Edwin L. Klingelhofer.
          294 + xiv pp., 15.24 x 22.86 cm
     Includes index.
     ISBN 0-89603-225-6
     1. Allergy—Popular works. 2. Allergy—Prevention. 3. Allergy—Environmental sapects. I. Klingelhofer, E. L. (Ed L.) II. Title.
     RC584.G453   1992
     616.97'05—dc20   91-45417
                                                                        CIP

10 9 8 7 6 5 4 3

Preface

The world is full of naturally occurring and human-made substances capable of causing troublesome reactions in susceptible individuals. These reactions can be roughly classified according to:

- the bodily systems they affect
- how long they last
- the ease with which they can be treated
- whether they are allergic, hypersensitive, or toxic in origin
- how rapidly they develop following exposure to the trigger.

This book deals with the many thousands of these materials capable of provoking fast-appearing, relatively short-lived, and usually manageable allergic or hypersensitive reactions in the respiratory, gastrointestinal, or cutaneous (skin) systems of the human body. It tells you:

- what forms the symptoms take
- the environments in which they tend to turn up
- what their possible causes are and how you can go about identifying the one or ones responsible for your condition

v

- the steps you can take to avoid exposure entirely or significantly reduce its risk
- what forms of treatment are most likely to eliminate or control your symptoms.

The book does not cover reactions to substances—usually human-made ones—that cause severe, stubborn, debilitating damage. Here the culprits are likely to be chemicals linked to cancer, silicosis, asbestosis, and other forms of grave damage that are thought to develop after prolonged exposure to some causative agent, more often than not in the workplace. Likewise, it only touches incidentally on the two major causes of chronic and crippling disease in our society —tobacco and alcohol—whose dangers, unhappily, are as well known as they are ignored.

It also has nothing to say about "recreational" drugs whose risks and remedies are sufficiently familiar to anyone able to read the front page of a daily newspaper or follow a television news program. Nor does it dwell on vague, ill-defined, scientifically undocumented, modish symptoms or syndromes that are often, but unpersuasively, attributed to allergy or hypersensitivity to food, drink, exposure to chemicals, and the like. An example of this class of ailment is Tension-Fatigue Syndrome, said to be the result of allergic or hypersensitive reactions to food elements in the diet. There is no solid evidence to bear out this linkage.

Even with these constraints, we believe that the allergic conditions we discuss here are nearly as ubiquitous as the common cold and cause as much distress, adding up to as great an economic and human cost as any other group of illnesses that we might have chosen to write about. Asthma, for instance, one of the major allergic diseases—and certainly the most frightening of them—is the main reason for chronic school absences among children and contributes significantly and needlessly to poor school performance and stunted social, physical, and intellectual development in some of its sufferers.

Hay fever triggered by pollens, molds, dust, and other airborne particles causes acute and largely avoidable physical discomfort, absence from work or school, and impairs performance or severely restricts activity in the millions of Americans who suffer from it.

To these allergy sufferers add the other millions who are sensitive to certain foods or food additives—berries, eggs, legumes, shellfish, preservatives, dyes, walnuts—or who break out in a rash when they touch things as wildly disparate and commonplace as toilet soap, poison ivy, nickel-plated watchbands, fabric softener, or "No Carbon Required" paper. Throw in the additional legions who develop unwanted and sometimes dangerous side reactions to such common medications as aspirin or antibiotics. And don't forget the hordes who are made acutely uncomfortable by tobacco smoke, pollutants, fumes, and even perfumes and scents. Then there are the unlucky ones who develop serious reactions to insect stings or bites, or even, in some cases, are made ill by breathing in particles of insect bodies or the compounds used to get rid of them. Joining them are the unfortunates who react to animal dander from cats, dogs, horses, and even birds.

These triggers of allergy or irritation can turn up any place, any time.

The information we have systematically compiled in this book cannot be found in any other single source. It can help you and your family greatly. Its suggestions about health care reflect the best and most up-to-date medical information and opinion available. As with all medical advice, however, cases—and therefore treatments—may vary.

It is not intended to be an alternative to or substitute for your own doctor's recommendations. In particular, the treatment of severe, protracted, or stubborn symptoms or the use of *any* medication should be undertaken only after consultation with your own physician. The authors and publisher therefore disclaim any responsibility for consequences resulting from following the advice or procedures set forth here.

The book strives for completeness and clarity. We have tried to steer away from medical jargon and to assure that our contents are as accurate and comprehensive as we are humanly able to make them. To render the text more readable, reports of actual individual case histories, drawn from our experience, appear throughout.

The book is divided into six parts:

- Part 1 tells you how substances that invade your body act to make you sick.
- Part 2 describes the various allergic or irritant reactions in detail and says something about their prevalence, persistence, severity, and manageability.
- Part 3 offers detailed procedures you can follow to identify the cause of your symptoms and sketches some general strategies you can follow to avoid them.
- Part 4 deals with the various carriers of allergic or irritant reactions—food, drink, the air you breathe,

the things you touch or are touched by—and catalogs the substances capable of producing symptoms in susceptible individuals.

- Part 5—the heart of the book—tells you how to go about creating allergen or irritant-safe environments at home, out-of-doors, at school or on the job, in health care settings, or while traveling. It also offers a chapter on the so-called Sick Building Syndrome, an interesting and tricky condition that seems to be an unanticipated outgrowth of the move to build energy efficient structures, complicated by the growing use of synthetic or chemically treated materials in their construction and decor, and exacerbated by human suggestibility. The seven chapters in Part 5 are pivotal because *the first and, by all odds, the most effective tactic in the care of allergic or hypersensitive reactions is to avoid their cause.*

- Part 6, the last section of the book, identifies sources of help—and tells you how to go about lining up that help—from both public or private sources, should it be needed. The book ends with a set of appendixes that list allergens and irritants and provides other information that will be useful to you in developing strategies for coping with your problem.

Like all other writers on medical subjects we are indebted, first of all, to the researchers and practitioners who, over the millenia, have brought us to our present state of knowledge. Beyond them, and more particularly, we owe thanks to the Hornet Foundation of California State University, Sacramento, which generously provided funds to support the research that went into this endeavor. We also very much appreciate and acknowledge the help of Dr. Paul Davis in preparing the figures and of Drs. Christopher Chang, Georges Halpern, Bruce Ryhal, and Ronald Ruhl for their careful proofreading and critique. We especially want to thank Nikki Rojo, whose incomparable secretarial and administrative skills brought the manuscript into being.

Whatever flaws, errors, or shortcomings may yet be found here are ours alone.

M. Eric Gershwin, MD
Edwin L. Klingelhofer, PhD

Contents

xi

PART I

HOW WHAT YOU EAT, DRINK, TOUCH, OR BREATHE CAN MAKE YOU SICK

CHAPTER 1

Allergens and Irritants

What They Are, How They Can Make You Sick, and the Sicknesses They Trigger

Almost any substance that the human body can come into contact with is capable of making someone, somewhere, sick. Foods, pollens, smoke, fumes, dust, medications, plants, herbicides, pesticides, fungicides, and the thousands of chemicals that are a part of our environment are all capable, in susceptible individuals, of provoking reactions that range from trivial to life-threatening to life-denying.

These reactions usually show up first in the respiratory, gastrointestinal, or cutaneous systems of the body—the lungs, the airways and passages leading to them, the digestive system, or the skin. Why these systems? Because they are the ones that directly interface with the environment outside of the human body, and afford the paths by which foreign substances are introduced into it. These transactions with our environment are necessary, of course—we must have food, liquids, and air to sustain life.

These life-sustaining elements can, and frequently do, carry materials that cause sickness. The troubles caused by these invading substances can be roughly classified into allergic, irritant or intolerant, toxic, or immunosuppressant reactions.

3

Allergic Reactions

Paul Langerhans (1847–1888) was a famous Prussian physician, a Professor of Pathology, and one of the most influential figures in medicine in his time. One of his contributions was discovery of the pancreatic cells that make insulin and are destroyed in people who have diabetes, cells now known as the "islets of Langerhans." Langerhans had a son who had been exposed to diphtheria at school—in those days usually a fatal disease. To prevent diphtheria, children exposed to the disease were given shots of a serum made from the blood of horses. This horse serum vaccination often kept the exposed child from developing the deadly symptoms. The Langerhans boy was given the horse serum inoculation. Sadly, he was exquisitely allergic to horses, and so immediately went into shock and died. His case became widely known and led eventually to the development of the concept of allergy and acute allergic reaction.

Most people have an idea of what an allergy is. And almost certainly they know someone who suffers, or even themselves suffer from allergic diseases such as eczema, hay fever, or asthma. Unfortunately, the word allergy has come to take on broad and inaccurate connotations, so that it is now applied loosely and often inappropriately to many conditions that are not strictly allergic, or even physical in nature. You may not like your boss, or getting up early, or rock music, but saying that you are "allergic" to those circumstances of life destroys the meaning of the term.

Whenever she ingests alcohol in any form Lois develops flushing and experiences short-lived difficulties in breathing. However, her symptoms are not an allergic reaction; she is simply intolerant of alcohol.[1]

In Chapter 2, we will explain what happens in the body to produce a true allergic reaction and then will enumerate the forms that these reactions take.

Many people do not realize that an allergen, the material that induces an allergy, is but one specific chemical in a broad variety of classes of chemicals that can influence our bodies. We say "chemicals" because, in a sense, everything in the world is chemical, including the human body and all its reactions or responses. To be truly an "allergen" the substance must be capable of triggering the production of a special antibody called IgE. It may help the reader appreciate the complexity of allergic reactions by pointing out that, when the blood of an allergic person is injected into a normal (non-allergic) volunteer, the allergy itself is transferred for several days. This cross-reaction is called the PK reaction after the names of the people who discovered it, Carl Prausnitz and Heinz Kustner. Kustner was very allergic to fish. Prausnitz, a non-allergic person, collected blood from his colleague, Kustner, and injected it into himself. For a period of time thereafter, Prausnitz, who received the injection, showed a local allergic reaction to fish.

---

[1]In this and all succeeding reports of individual cases, the names and many details have been changed to protect the identities of the persons concerned.

Irritant or Intolerant Reactions

In addition to allergies, there are other types or classes of bodily reactions to chemicals. One of these classes is that involved in the response to irritants. We have all had experience with irritants.

> Pat works in a large office in downtown Pittsburgh. She has no known allergies and is in generally good health. However, she is very sensitive to tobacco smoke and exposure provokes a dry cough and makes her eyes tear. Pat is not really allergic to tobacco smoke, although her symptoms are much like those seen in allergic diseases, since no IgE is produced. She is simply more sensitive to the smoke than most people. For Pat, regardless of the label hung on the cause, the result is the same—she gets sick. However, in her case, the smoke is an irritant and her reaction is not a true allergy.

You may wonder why it makes any difference at all whether your problem is an allergic or an irritant reaction. In either instance you will first try to deal with it by removing the offending material from your environment. However, as we shall discuss more completely in Chapter 2, in the case of an allergy your physician will usually go on to prescribe medication to make you better. In addition, the cause of a true allergy—pollen for instance—is often very difficult to remove from the environment, so that treatment is two-pronged, aimed at both removal of the allergen to the extent possible and at the treatment of symptoms. The treatment for an irritant reaction to, say, cigaret smoke is much simpler. Avoid or get rid of the cause—declare your home or workplace a smoke-free zone.

There is a myriad of possible irritants and more keep turning up all the time. Table 1 lists some of the more common ones, Later on, in Part 4, we will discuss each of these irritants in more detail and spell out strategies for their removal or avoidance in air, water, and food, and at home, school, work, or in other environments.

Table 1

Common Causes of Irritant Reactions

1. Tobacco smoke	9. Paints
2. Smog	10. Perfumes/incense
3. Ozone	11. Dyes
4. Formaldehyde	12. Paper/pulp products
5. Ammonia	13. Chlorinated chemicals
6. Sulfur dioxide	14. Pesticides/herbicides
7. Gasoline/oil fumes	15. Soaps/detergents
8. Glues, pastes	16. Fungicides

Toxic Reactions

Toxins cause reactions quite different from those produced by allergens or irritants. Toxin means poison. The word poison usually conjures a vision of somebody slipping something fast-acting and lethal into somebody else's drink and being found out, a few corpses later, by Perry Mason or some other super-sleuth. However, many toxic chemicals exert effects that are delayed for years—even decades—before their effects show up.

George worked as a welder in Navy shipyards
during World War II. He routinely handled and
breathed in asbestos. Although the government
and the manufacturer knew of the dangers of asbestos, they never shared this knowledge with
George or his coworkers. Thirty years later George
developed a severe cough and a pain in his chest.
His doctor found fluid in his lung and a cancer in
his chest called a mesothelioma. George died
within months of the discovery of his cancer, as
have tens of thousands of other people who had
been exposed to asbestos 10 to 40 years earlier.
It took three decades for the asbestos to do its
dirty work in George's case.

Most people have heard about the dangers of
asbestos and the hazards it presents to workers in
the insulation and fire-retardant industries. But how
many realize that asbestos was used in the majority
of buildings—homes, schools, offices, and factories—
built in this country throughout the 20th century? The
removal of asbestos poses special risks and must be
undertaken by carefully trained workers who wear
special equipment. Yet, in 1989, a news story surfaced
charging that workers involved in the construction of
the famous Trump Tower in Manhattan worked with
asbestos without having had any training in its safe
handling and without observing any of the manda-
tory safety precautions.

Table 2 lists some of the more notorious toxins
associated with cancer and a variety of other diseases.
This list can only grow longer, what with the relent-
less introduction of new products into all aspects of
the home and working environments—products whose

Table 2
Materials and Chemicals Associated with Cancer

1. Asbestos	8. Benzene/other solvents
2. Paints/stains	9. Petrochemicals (gasoline, oils)
3. X-radiation	10. Arsenic
4. Tobacco smoke	11. Ashes/charcoal
5. Some food dyes	12. Saccharine
6. Alcohol	13. Selenium
7. Pesticides	14. Herbicides

long-term effects on humans are unstudied and will be, if past experience is any guide, damaging. You have the right to and should demand to know what you are being exposed to. You have the right to clean air and water. And you should keep in mind that your government and American industry have not always been forthright in informing you of risks.

Jack is a Vietnam vet. During the war he was assigned the job of handling Agent Orange. Jack, like many veterans of that unhappy conflict, died of cancer when he was only 39. Even now the government and the American scientific establishment does not know, or is unwilling to disclose, the long-term health implications of exposure to Agent Orange. Though both American and Australian studies suggest that Agent Orange may have been harmless, there continues to be controversy over the long-term toxicity of the herbicide.

Almost every one of us, every day, comes into contact with toxins used as herbicides, pesticides, preservatives, or food colors. Who has the knowledge to say that a new preservative will not end up by poisoning us—or our unborn offspring—in 30 year's time?

More than a century ago it was discovered that bladder and testicular cancer was very common in chimney sweepers in England. This landmark discovery was the first of many associations of exposure to certain materials in the workplace and the later development of cancer.

> Like many of her compatriots, Inga, a Finnish office worker, loves smoked fish. And Inga, like many another person living in cultures that consume large quantities of smoked fish products, has developed gastric cancer.

One has to wonder how many other cancers are associated with things we eat, breathe, or touch that have not yet been identified as carcinogens.

The growing realization that more and more chemicals have invaded our environment and the discovery that some of them have serious negative impacts on the health of humans and other species has brought about a significant change in public attitudes toward chemicals.

For many years one of the largest of the chemical manufacturers strenuously proclaimed that its mission was to provide better things for better living through chemistry. After Love Canal, Bhopal, the spill that contaminated the entire reach of the Rhine river, and the proliferation of toxic dump sites all over the globe, chemical companies no longer do much advertizing and seem to be reticent about proclaiming the nature of their activities. In a sense, the pendulum of public opinion has gone from the extreme of believing that chemistry held the prospect of opening the good life to all to the opposite extreme of viewing it as a shop of horrors.

There is little doubt that chemistry has been of enormous immediate benefit to much of the world's population—it has also imperiled the environment and launched ecological crises or disasters of unprecedented magnitude and gravity. DDT in the food chain, herbicides leaching out of the fields and killing plant and animal life in lakes and streams, acid rain, the breached ozone layer, the greenhouse effect—all trace back to the innocent, joyous, indiscriminate, heedless use of chemicals. Yet, completely avoiding chemicals is and always has been an impossibility. The consumption of "organic" foods is rising sharply, for example, and we agree that farmers should use as few chemicals as possible in their farming. However, it is worth noting that plants have their own ways of protecting themselves against insects and other threats, largely by themselves producing chemicals. Some of these plant-produced chemicals may well prove to be worse—more toxic—than manufactured pesticides.

The role commercially available chemicals ought to play in our lives is hard to decide. Such a determination calls for an open mind and resistance to the blandishments of the extremists at both poles of the dispute about the place of chemicals. Chemicals, like poverty, are always with us. Perhaps a solution is to be found through education and the development of a mindset that emphasizes cultivation of the patience to weigh long-term effects, puts environmental considerations before profits, and places prime value on conservation as opposed to consumerism.

Table 3

Drugs and Chemicals in Common Use
That Can Destroy Blood Cells

Drugs

1. Phenylbutazone (antiarthritic)
2. Chloramphenicol (antibiotic)
3. Propylthiouracil (used in thyroid treatment)
4. Methotrexate (used for treatment of severe asthma, arthritis, and for cancer)
5. Gold salts (antiarthritic)
6. Cytoxan (used for lupus and for cancer)
7. Imuran (used for lupus and for cancer)
8. Other—theoretically, *any* drug can produce a cytotoxic reaction in a susceptible person

Chemicals

1. Petrochemicals
2. Paints
3. Arsenic
4. Pesticides/herbicides
5. Benzene/solvents

Immunosuppressant Reactions

Finally, there is a fourth and last reaction to chemicals and drugs. These reactions are the result of immunosuppression. In order to survive, we have to be able to fight infections and to make white blood cells. Yet there are chemicals in the environment, and drugs that are used to treat persons with such diseases as cancer and arthritis, that can reduce the body's ability to fight infections. These compounds are called immunosuppressants. They are considered "cytotoxic," that is, they kill cells. Your doctor is acutely aware of the perilous side effects carried by these drugs and, in most cases, they are prescribed by a specialist who is well-trained in their use. Some of the chemicals that can produce immunosuppression are listed in Table 3. Please note that, on rare occasions, any drug can inadvertently produce peculiar or idiosyncratic reactions that can lead to immunosuppression and death.

> Bill was troubled with chronic and painful cramps in his legs. He saw his family doctor, who prescribed a drug called phenylbutazone. Bill was not warned that a small but significant number of individuals can develop immunosuppression, a disease called agranulocytosis, from taking phenylbutazone. Bill found out the hard way and died of pneumonia.

Phenylbutazone is not used very often any more; we believe it should not be used at all.

As a patient, you should never forget that you have the right to ask your doctor what the side effects of your medications may be. All drugs have side effects, but some are safer than others. The best advice we can give is to encourage you not to use any drug at all if your condition is self-limiting—likely to get better on its own. Don't give your cold to Contac® in the first place or to any of the scores of other cold "remedies." They don't get rid of the cold, which will go away on its own eventually. In the second place they can and often do carry troublesome side-effects that are worse than the cold symptoms.

> Joan had a cold and saw her doctor. Joan's doctor uses antibiotics on everyone for almost everything. He prescribed a drug called chloramphenicol. Joan's cold got better almost immedi-

ately. In fact it would have gotten better just as fast without the antibiotic which, like all antibiotics, is ineffective against viruses, but does help to convince patients that the doctor is doing something. Two months later, Joan's body stopped making blood cells, a rare complication of chloramphenicol, and she later died, a terrible price to have to pay for the placebo effect.

Chloramphenicol has been removed from common use, thank God! However, Joan's condition, aplastic anemia, can be induced by many materials, including fumes from paints and petrochemicals, as well as by drugs. Few of us are aware of this, and very little testing of the physical/physiological consequences of exposure to potential immunosuppressants is ever done.

There are virtually limitless ways by which what you eat, drink, touch, or breathe can make you sick. It is a dangerous world out there, but one that can be made safer for you and yours through thoughtful, prudent, systematic study and analysis. In this book we will teach you how to do this by supplying the information and skills you need and showing you how to develop the attitudes that will foster this approach. In the end you will know the right questions to ask and will be able to face your environment more knowingly and confidently.

Points to Remember

In this chapter we have sketched the several kinds of reactions—allergic, hypersensitivity, toxic, immunosuppressant—that can be triggered by substances you may encounter in your various activities. In the rest of the book, however, we will focus more sharply on allergic and irritant-caused symptoms. Though a given substance can provoke either an allergic or an irritant reaction, the form the reaction takes depends on the susceptibility of the individual. Thus, it is important to establish the cause and nature of a reaction in order to treat it effectively and economically.

PART 2

ALLERGIC
AND IRRITANT REACTIONS

CHAPTER 2

What Allergens Are
and Why People Have Allergies

Their Prevalence, Persistence, Severity,
and Manageability

An allergen is any substance that triggers the production by the human immune system of a special antibody called Immunoglobulin E—IgE for short. IgE is one of five types of antibodies that we all make—IgG, IgM, IgA, IgD, and IgE. IgE is the antibody that responds to those materials or foreign substances that impinge on us from the outside world. It is manufactured in special cells along the inside of the tubes that deliver the air we breathe and along the intestine that digests the food we eat. In short, IgE production is our own immune response to things eaten, breathed, or (in certain instances) touched.

Virtually all mammals make IgE when they are infected with worms. Researchers believe that the IgE antibody evolved so that worms could be killed and prevented from causing infection. Though worms have largely ceased to be a problem for humans in Western society, all of us continue to produce IgE antibodies. People whose immune systems manufacture relatively more IgE in response to allergens are the ones prone to develop allergies.

The ability to make large amounts of IgE is inherited and clearly runs in families. Thus, if your mother or brother has allergies, then you are more likely to develop allergies yourself than if they were free of symptoms. The rule of inheritability is not absolute, however; allergies do appear in individuals who have no family history of allergy. And some individuals with very strong family histories escape having allergies altogether.

Tracy remembers the first time she heard the word "atopic." When she was five years old, during one of many visits to her pediatrician, she was given a cup of Mountain Dew, a soft drink, to satisfy her thirst. Within minutes she had developed a rash all over her body. Her mother showed it to the pediatrician who promptly added the beverage to a very long list of things Tracy was allergic to. She went on to say that Tracy was one of the most atopic children she had ever seen. Both of Tracy's parents also have allergies.

Sally is one of five children. Her brothers and sisters all carry inhalers and seem to be constantly sneezing, wheezing, or scratching. Someone in the house always seems to be sick with an allergy of one sort or another. Sally's parents are not allergic at all and Sally, who seems to have inherited her parents' resistance, doesn't understand how her sibs can be so vulnerable.

How Common Are Allergies?

Allergies are found in up to 10% of children. The allergies may range from mild hay fever to life-threat-

Table 4

The Most Common Allergens[1]

Allergen	Americans affected, %
1. Plant pollen and wood products	15
2. Animal dander—especially cat	5
3. Molds	2
4. Dust and dust mites	5
5. Antibiotics, including penicillin	2–10
6. Milk and milk products	1–3
7. Shrimp	0.5–2
8. Nuts	0.5–1

[1]Though this is a list of the most common allergens, we remind our readers that theoretically any substance is capable of inducing an allergy. Triggers may range from the prescription drugs listed in Table 5 to the glue on the back of a postage stamp!

ening asthma. In *Conquering Your Child's Allergies*[1] we discuss childhood allergies in detail. For most individuals the cause of an allergy can be established through a good history taken by your doctor, supplemented by the use of food, blood, or skin tests and, where necessary, an elimination diet. Some of the more common allergies and their prevalence are named in Table 4.

The complaints caused by the allergens listed in Table 4 are commonplace and can usually be diagnosed confidently. More difficult to identify, however, are the many unknown constituents found in food. We are still living in the Dark Ages when it comes to under-

[1]See Gershwin, M. Eric and Klingelhofer, Edwin L., *Conquering Your Child's Allergies,* Addison-Wesley Publishing Company, Reading, Massachusetts, 1989.

Table 5

Drugs Frequently Associated with Allergic Reactions

Drug	Use	Reaction
Penicillin[1]	Antibiotic	Rash, wheezing, hives, anaphylaxis
Sulfonamides	Antibiotics	Rash, wheezing, hives, Stevens-Johnson syndrome, anaphylaxis
Lasix	Diuretic	Rash
Motrin[2]	Antiarthritic	Rash, wheezing
Warfarin	Anticlotting	Rash
Novocaine	Local anesthetic	Rash, anaphylaxis

[1]There are many drugs similar to penicillin that can induce the same problems, e.g., ampicillin. If you are allergic to one penicillin you are usually allergic to all types of penicillin.

[2]Other antiarthritic drugs, such as aspirin, naproxen, and indomethacin, can cause the same problem.

standing food allergy, the accurate diagnosis of which remains one of the most difficult problems in medicine. Finally, one should never forget that drugs—prescription or over-the-counter—often cause allergic reactions. The more common offenders are listed in Table 5.

How Persistent Are Allergies?

Allergies last for life. Even though the severity of symptoms may diminish or appear to vanish, the allergic tendency persists and can still be detected when rigorous testing is done. Children do not outgrow their allergies; rather, they outgrow their pediatricians.

Joy is allergic to soy sauce. She knows she must avoid soy beans all of her life and has not slipped up in 35 years. However, at a New Year's party she is offered a cup of home-made sweet and sour soup containing soy sauce. Because it had been so long since she had suffered a reaction she decides to take a chance. She nearly dies of breathing difficulties that appear within minutes.

Laurie, a busy University Professor, has had a lifelong allergy to shrimp. She recently flew to Chicago to attend a conference and, because the plane was overbooked, she was selected to move up to First Class. There she chose the lasagna for lunch. To her dismay her tongue began to swell and hives developed almost as soon as she took her first bite of the pasta. She poked through the lasagna and found that it contained a few tiny shrimp. Afterwards Laurie wished that she had stayed in the tourist section and eaten the Chicken Tetrazzini. That way she might not have spent her first day in Chicago in the emergency room.

Severity of Allergies

The severity of an allergy varies greatly between people and from allergen to allergen. There are many surprises out there.

Martha Ellis and her husband, Herb, both have ragweed-triggered hay fever. Martha's symptoms are very mild; some sneezing, a runny nose, and tearing of the eyes that she controls with over-the-counter antihistamines. Herb, on the other hand, has to take elaborate environmental precautions and starts a course of prescription preventive medications well in advance of the ragweed season. If he fails to carry out these precautionary steps, as he has on a couple of occasions, he winds up in the emergency room with a violent case of hay fever complicated by a life-threatening asthmatic attack.

A few unlucky individuals develop allergic reactions to triggers that are innocuous for almost everyone else.

Flo invariably broke out in acute hives following sex with her husband. She saw her doctor about the problem and, although she was vividly aware of the temporal relationship between intercourse and her hives, she was too embarrassed to tell her doctor. Needless to say, the doctor, who was not a mind reader, did not make the connection. He prescribed antihistamines and for the next few years, Flo spent a small fortune on drugs and a lot of time suffering from their after-effects when relief from the distressing symptoms was only a condom away.

The list of materials that can induce true allergic reactions is continually growing.

Art is a health food nut. He spends over $50 a week buying vitamins, amino acids, and all sorts of building blocks that he takes according to a schedule that is nearly as complicated as the invasion plans for D-day. Art believes he is being healthy. In fact he is endangering his life because one of the things he takes is an amino acid called L-tryptophan. Not long after starting on it he developed wracking muscle pains. Tests showed that he has thousands of eosinophils in his blood and muscle. This disease, called *eosinophilic fasciitis*, developed in an unexpectedly large number of people in the Fall of 1989. We do not yet know whether it is an allergy; the overload of eosinophils suggests it may well be. We *are* convinced that somehow this health food, L-tryptophan, is responsible for Art's painful and disabling symptoms. Health foods can be dangerous to your health.

Allergic reactions can involve any one or a combination of bodily systems and, as we have noted, can range in severity from a minor and transitory annoyance to chronic and potentially life-threatening episodes.

Manageability of Allergies

In most instances allergies can be managed effectively by combining avoidance tactics with appropriate medication where necessary.

The first step in management is to identify whatever it is that is triggering your symptoms. If you do not already know this (most people have a pretty good idea about the cause of their symptoms), Chapter 4 offers strategies you can adopt to pin down the cause of your reaction. Once the allergen affecting you is identified, you can act to banish it from your life. Procedures for accomplishing this are spelled out in Chapter 5 and Parts 4 and 5. For instance, if your trigger is a particular food, you should pay close attention to Chapters 6 and 10; if it is an airborne substance, Chapter 7 and the chapters in Part 5 that are relevant to your situation—the how, when, where, and why of your symptoms—will be instructive.

If you cannot nail down your nemesis, or if it is so persistent and widespread that you are unable to avoid contact with it (this is true for a few such allergens as pollens and air pollutants and of asthma induced by respiratory infections, for instance), then you will need to seek help. The various sources of help are identified in Part 6. Where allergies are concerned, you should probably start with your family doctor and, if he or she fails to help you, consult with an allergist certified by the American Academy of Allergy and Immunology. (A substantial number of physicians make a business of treating patients with allergies. Unless they are board-certified specialists in allergy, they may not have the up-to-date information and knowledge of the special techniques needed to help you manage your symptoms efficiently and economically.)

Your family doctor or allergist, after taking a careful history, may subject you to additional tests to find out whether your reaction is, in fact, allergic and to pin down whatever is causing it. Following diagnosis, you may then have medications prescribed or, in some instances, may begin a series of shots designed to desensitize you to the effects of the allergen. Allergy shots are administered more or less routinely to individuals who suffer severe reactions to bee stings or who have chronic, stubborn hay fever. In Chapter 14 we have listed precautions you ought to take if you are given allergy shots.

If medication is prescribed for your condition, two words of caution. First, take pains to learn about its possible side effects from the doctor or from the *Physician's Desk Reference* before using the drug. If side effects appear, notify your doctor immediately.

Second, be sure to follow the doctor's instructions for taking medication exactly as ordered. Failure to take drugs as prescribed is commonplace, and is often associated with poor control of symptoms or, less often, serious rebound of symptoms, sometimes with fatal consequences.

Points to Remember

An allergy is a specific and complex reaction to a substance that invades the human body. Allergic reactions are, in a sense, the result of an overreaction of the body's immune system to the invader.

It is estimated that as many as one in five Americans will suffer from some form of allergic disease during their lifetime.

Susceptibility to allergies is clearly inherited, although the specific mechanism and the likelihood of any given individual developing symptoms is not precisely known. This susceptibility to allergy is quite durable and persists for the sufferer's life.

Allergic symptoms range in severity from occasional mildly uncomfortable short-lived episodes to chronic, disabling, and life-threatening disease. The list of substances known to provoke allergies is constantly growing, although a relatively small number of foods and food additives, airborne particles, and materials coming in contact with the skin account for most cases.

Allergies, regardless of their severity, can almost always be managed effectively by combining appropriate medication with strategies aimed at avoiding exposure to the trigger.

CHAPTER 3

Irritants and
Acquired Defects in Immunity

*Their Effects, Prevalence,
Severity, and Manageabliity*

Substances inhaled, touched, or ingested can cause allergic reactions, but you don't have to be allergic to have something in your environment make you sick. You can react directly to a substance without involving your immune system and releasing histamine. As a matter of fact, given the multitude of contaminants in the environment in 20th century America, the number of people with irritant-induced illness greatly exceeds those with allergy-triggered complaints.

> Barbara can smell a cigaret a mile away—or at least she says so. For virtually all of her life she has developed a cough, often accompanied by nasal congestion, whenever she encounters second-hand tobacco smoke. She is now 25. She finds wry satisfation in the knowledge that the harmfulness of second-hand smoke has only recently been established. As a child she was told she was *allergic* to tobacco smoke—the only "allergy" she had. She is robustly healthy unless she is near a

29

smoker, in an airplane with smokers, or otherwise exposed to tobacco smoke. Since it does not
trigger the chain of reactions associated with allergic illness and her symptoms clear up as soon
as the smoke is removed, it is simply an irritant
in Barbara's case.

An irritant, when encountered by a sensitive person, acts to provoke a reaction directly; the form the
reaction takes depends on the organ of the body affected. If you walk through a patch of poison oak and are
susceptible to it, expect a rash to develop directly and
quickly; if you can't handle green pepper and inadvertently ingest some with your stir-fry, gastric distress will not be far behind; if you can't stand tobacco
smoke and your cigar-smoking uncle lights up a huge
stogie after the family Thanksgiving dinner, are you
ready for the coughing and wheezing?
     Since nothing about allergy or sensitivity is
simple, there is an important qualifier to add here. In
the case of allergic individuals, the amount of an
irritant necessary to provoke a reaction may be much,
much lower than it is in normal, non-allergic people.
One often encounters instances of this lowered thresh-
old of excitability.

> Terry has had respiratory allergies and asthma
> all of her life. Whenever she is exposed to tobacco
> smoke (and a long list of other chemicals) she
> quickly finds it necessary to use her inhaler. She
> does not even smell the tobacco, but her airways
> clearly know it is there and the most minute ex-
> posure is enough to stimulate her bronchospasm
> and start her to wheezing.

The physical effects of irritants are much the same as those of allergens; the same body systems are affected and the symptoms produced are quite similar. Allergic reactions appear after a period of sensitization—repeated exposure to the allergen—has occurred. In some instances it may take years for the allergic reaction to show up.

> Stan, an industrial arts teacher, retired with a disability. He supplements his pension doing home remodeling and repairs. Several jobs in a row entailed finishing (taping and texturing) sheet rock. After the second job he noticed that his hands were becoming sore and inflamed. During the third job, a much larger project, his hands developed a rash, swelled, cracked, and became extremely painful. He saw his family doctor, who referred him to a dermatologist, who diagnosed the problem as allergic contact dermatitis. The symptoms, he said, were brought on by chromate in the "mud" used for texturing the walls. "You sure about that, Doc?" Stan asked. "I've been around that stuff most of my life." "I'm sure," the doctor replied. "All that previous exposure was just getting you ready for retirement. Sensitizing you." The doctor treated Stan successfully, although his rash was extremely stubborn and slow to heal. Now Stan refuses to take on jobs that involve handling dry wall or concrete in any form.

Reactions to irritants, conversely, do not require the long sensitization period. Take a bite of your very first helping of sauteed shrimp. Boom! Hives all over the body.

Prevalence and Severity of Irritants and Irritant Reactions

In Table 6 we have listed some of the substances most well-known for their irritant properties and where they are discussed in this book. Irritants exist

Table 6
Common Irritants

Type of substance	Chapter where discussed
Airborne particles	7, 11, 12, 13, 15, 16
Bacteria	16
Pollens, dust and dust mites, mold and mildew spores	7, 11, 12, 13, 15
Animal dander	
Tobacco and other smoke	
Candle or incense fumes Smoke or fumes from heating devices	
Fumes from scent/cologne, Fumes from paints, mastics, varnishes, glues	7, 12
Pollutants (petrochemical) fumes, carbon monoxide, sulfur dioxide, ozone	7, 12, 13
Particles from household chemicals (powdered soaps, detergents, insecticides, insect repellents, various aerosol-driven sprays)	7, 12, 13
Substances touched or ingested	6, 9–16
Poisonous plants	9
Pesticides, herbicides, soaps, cleansers, fabric softeners, oven cleaners, shoe polish, cosmetics	9
	9, 12, 13, 15
Foods and food additives, medications	6, 10, 14, 15

in myriad; indeed, there probably exists someone who would react on exposure to nearly every substance in the world. Most adults, at some time or another in their lives, will suffer an adverse reaction to an irritant. Gastric distress, breathing difficulties, skin rashes—all are part of the fabric of life and irritants are likely to spawn most of these episodes.

Reactions to irritants develop relatively rapidly, are ordinarily shortlived, and respond promptly to treatment. So long as you distance yourself from the source of the difficulty, your symptoms will usually clear unaided, and moreover will not return provided you maintain sound avoidance tactics—good advice, but sometimes difficult to follow, especially where the irritant is ubiquitous.

However, in those instances when exposure to the offending substance continues, symptoms can become chronic and severe—even life-threatening. This is also true when an acute degree of sensitivity exists such that even the most brief and trivial encounter is capable of triggering an intense reaction. When this possibility exists, you must prepare for it by establishing emergency procedures and having appropriate medications available for immediate administration.

Manageability of Irritant Symptoms

As noted above, reactions to irritants are usually brief, mild, and treatable. If they are not, the best course of action for you to take is to consult your family physician, who will prescribe medications appropriate to the nature and location of the ailment. If the treatment seems to be ineffective or, as sometimes happens, appears to aggravate the symptoms, report this to the doctor and ask for a review of your situation and possible referral to a specialist—e.g., an allergist, dermatologist, internist, or pulmonary specialist. Though the symptoms may not be serious or distressing, they should not be allowed to persist to the point where you run the risk they will become chronic and acute.

A Note on the Avoidance of Irritants

The past twenty years or so have seen the emergence of a group of physicians who refer to themselves as clinical ecologists. These practitioners profess to treat what has variously been called "environmental illness," "multiple-chemical sensitivity," or "20th century disease." This specialty is not recognized by the American Medical Association; neither is the disease, whatever it is called, that they purport to treat.

These physicians contend that exposure to chemicals or sensitization by disease can make the susceptible individual hypersensitive to literally thousands of substances—even electromagnetic waves—substances that can then trigger a wide array of serious, disabling complaints.

One aspect of treatment offered by clinical ecologists is the design of environmentally shielded areas in which to live and work. Apart from being expensive, in our experience few if any individuals thrown into such environments have shown improvement. The world is full of chemicals. In fact, it is made up of chemicals, and purporting to create a chemical-free environment is an exercise in absurdity. It may be more instructive to keep Leon's case in mind when a diagnosis of multiple-chemical sensitivity is being put forth.

Leon devoutly believed that he had environmental illness. At work, at home, almost no matter where he was, he was subject to headaches, overwhelming fatigue, dizziness, weakness, and a helpless feeling of frustration. He was positive he was hypersensitive to something—chemicals, he thought—in his environment. Yet, on a vacation, while visiting his parents on the family farm, his symptoms improved. He attributed his flight into health to the clean, wholesome country air and environment, forgetting that farms are among the most chemically invaded, if not degraded, areas to be found. He discussed his improvement with his doctor who remained skeptical about Leon's hypothesis as to why he was better. The doctor probed Leon a bit further, and wound up by suggesting that a reduction in stress while Leon was away might have contributed to his bettered health. Leon admitted that he disliked his job and his boss and was terribly unhappy generally, but that he was stuck. He stayed with the job (and the symptoms stayed with Leon) for the next several years, but finally he was laid off by his employer. Even though he was unemployed, Leon's symptoms got better almost at once. He sought retraining, found a new job, and his symptoms did not return.

Our point here is that building a chemical-free environment is a forlorn hope. It is possible, with care, to avoid or effectively limit exposure to a modest list of known irritants, but if general hyperreactivity is claimed—or diagnosed—and blamed for a broad spectrum of vague and intractable symptoms, it may pay to look into the possible psychodynamics underlying the symptoms.

This is not to say that chemicals ought to be absolved of responsibility for symptoms. Far from it. New chemicals are entering our environment in waves, some without good reason, and many of them are quite capable of making you sick. Food dyes or preservatives are notable offenders; so are the pesticides and herbicides that increasingly invade our food chain, and are applied with such appalling carelessness by most users. If you have occasion to spread these dangerous chemicals, take pains to read and follow the directions scrupulously. Avoid bodily contact, use a mask, wear gloves, long sleeves, trousers, and apply only recommended amounts to the appropriate sites.

Another aspect of the chemical invasion has to do with medications. There has been a veritable explosion of medicines in the past quarter century. You might think that, being medicines, they are unqualifiedly good for you or, at least, won't hurt you. Think again! One of the major contributors to the rise in incidence of irritant symptoms has been the use (and abuse) of prescription and over-the-counter drugs. This is true because some of the newer drugs—antibiotics, for instance—are potent irritants in their own right. Aspirin ("...the wonder drug that works wonders") is responsible for a multitude of complaints, often inducing and intensifying respiratory and gastric symptoms, sometimes catastrophically. Other medications, notably topical antihistamines, will exacerbate some skin disorders, and anesthetics such as novocaine or benzocaine may provoke violent irritant reactions.

Even if medications do not in themselves present some risk, many of them contain artificial colors and preservatives that are known to be potent irritants. We are mystified why medications (or foods, come to that) seem to require added color to make them more acceptable to the consumer.

If you have a medication prescribed for you, insist that the physician (and pharmacist) specify exactly how and when it is to be taken, spell out possible reactions, provide a copy of the package insert that accompanies all drugs and enumerates possible side effects, and tell you what steps to take if the drug triggers a reaction or proves ineffectual.

And, while we are on the topic of drugs, remember that so-called recreational or psychotropic drugs—amphetamines, cocaine, alcohol, uppers, downers—have wide-ranging side effects that can wreak serious damage on the user. Don't use them!

Acquired Defects in Immunity

Our immune system begins to develop virtually from the time we are conceived. However, at birth much of it is still underdeveloped and during the first 6–12 months of life, we depend on maternal antibodies that have crossed the placenta to protect us from many infections. By the age of one year, the immune system becomes virtually our own. Early in life we are exposed for the first time to large numbers of viral and bacterial infections and our immune system "learns" to respond and to protect us from them. Thus, natural exposure to viruses and bacteria, as well as exposure by vaccination against the common childhood diseases, helps in the formation of an immune system that is amazingly complex and effective. This system fights infection by deploying a combination of lymphocytes and neutrophils (both are white blood cells), as well as antibodies. Powerful and resistant, it is capable of fighting an enormous number of potential infectious agents. This is known as the "systemic" immune system because it defends against infectious agents that reside within our bodies.

There is a second immune system known as "mucosal" immunity. This system defends against agents that enter through the nose (such as the air we breathe) and through the mouth (our food and drink). It relies on the same lymphocytes, neutrophils, and antibodies that characterize the systemic immunity system. However, it also depends greatly on a local form of "nonspecific" immunity. These are cells that line the airways and react against any inhaled infectious agents, as well as inhaled pollutants, that may come down the airways. They dispose of them by engulfing and digesting them in a very efficient process that amounts to a filtration device acting against particulate matter in the air.

There are many ways that this mucosal immune system can be suppressed. For example, exposure to tobacco smoke, to fumes, to dust, and even to cold air can impair the immune system. (This last cause of immune suppression—cold air—may be one reason why we are prone to develop colds when exposed to winter weather.)

Aging is another factor that evidently suppresses the immune system. An older individual gradually becomes less capable of producing antibodies than someone younger, which explains why older people find that they are more susceptible to colds and that it takes them longer to get rid of them. This trend is well-known to immunologists, who call it immuno-senescence or aging immunity.

There are also infections that compromise the effectiveness of the immune system. By far the most common is the acquired immune deficiency syndrome, or AIDS. In this disease a virus invades and kills thymus-derived lymphocytes, making it difficult, if not impossible, for patients to ward off attacks by every-day infectious agents, especially viruses and a rare protozoal disease called pneumocystis. There are a variety of transient defects in immunity that occur during viral infections. For example, before measles vaccination was widespread, it was not uncommon for a serious pneumonia to occur in a person with measles. In fact, before measles vaccination is given, children undergo skin testing for tuberculosis—to be certain they are not harboring the tuberculosis bacterium. If the TB bacterium is present, the measles serum may suppress the immune system and activate tuberculo-sis. Influenza may be another example of a viral ill-ness that can transiently affect the immune system.

There are, in addition, certain acquired diseases called autoimmune diseases, in which the body, in effect, turns against itself and makes antibodies that attack its own tissues and (in some instances) its own immune system. The best studied of these diseases is systemic lupus erythematosus—lupus, as it is com-

Table 7
Causes of Defects in the Immune System

I.   Chemical/environmental
     A. Tobacco
     B. Other pollutants
     C. Cold air
     D. Petrochemicals
     E. Silica
II. Infections
     A. "Permanent"—acquired immune deficiency
        syndrome (AIDS)
     B. Transient—measles, influenza, other viruses
III. Autoimmune or connective tissue diseases
     A. Systemic lupus erythematosus
     B. Scleroderma
     C. Sjögren's syndrome
     D. Rheumatoid arthritis
IV. Cancers of the immune system
     A. Leukemia
     B. Lymphoma
     C. Hodgkin's disease
     D. Multiple myeloma
V.   Age
     A. Generally older than 65

---

monly called. This illness has nothing whatsoever to
do with allergies, but there is some reason to suspect
that lupus may be partially induced by factors in the
environment. It has been shown that the administration of certain mercury compounds can readily induce
a lupus-like disease in otherwise healthy animals. The
origin of lupus remains obscure and research is now
underway to determine whether there are chemicals
that may be responsible for its onset. Diseases etio-
logically similar to lupus are listed in Table 7.

Finally, there are several malignancies that compromise the immune system, including certain cancers—lymphoma, Hodgkin's disease, leukemia, and multiple myeloma. These are unique problems whose causes are unknown, but there remains concern that some of them may be induced by chemical exposure. A great deal of research is needed on this matter.

Points to Remember

In this chapter we have noted that substances that are inhaled, touched, or ingested can cause reactions without involving your immune system. In fact, the number of people with irritation or chemically induced illness greatly exceeds those who have true allergic complaints.

Much more research is needed before we understand the impact these chemicals have on the immune system and it is important to distinguish true irritant reactions from those that may be psychologically based. One should be wary of the so-called "clinical ecologists" unless they can back up their diagnoses of "environmental illness" with data. There is no credible evidence that the clinical ecologists' fabrication of environmentally shielded areas is an effective measure. Some complaints blamed on irritants—or allergens—may be psychogenic in origin.

Finally, we note that the immune system responds vigorously to a variety of infectious agents. Defects in the system can result from infection, exposure to certain chemicals, and the onset of autoimmune diseases. Specific cancers can also compromise the immune system and increase susceptibility to infection.

PART 3

LOCATING CAUSES FOR AND AVOIDING ALLERGIC OR IRRITANT REACTIONS

CHAPTER 4

Strategies for Locating the Causes of Allergic or Irritant Reactions

Pinning down the cause or causes of your allergic or irritant reaction is the vital first step toward managing or controlling your symptoms. This can be a difficult and frustrating task, and we urge you to be patient and objective in doing so. Avoid falling for the seductive promises of speedy cures or control put forward by a small number of unscrupulous physicians and other health care providers. Keep a "Show me!" attitude; ask yourself whether any of the claims advanced are truly believable.

Beth didn't much like doctors, nor did she like waiting for appointments. She had already consulted several doctors, without result, about a lifelong problem with headaches when a friend suggested that her headaches might be allergic in origin. Initially skeptical, she succumbed to the argument when told there was a new doctor in town who practiced "environmental" medicine and "orthomolecular science." She was particularly impressed by the size of his newspaper ad and his convenient location in a shopping mall. The doctor could see her almost immediately and virtually guaranteed a cure. Several months and sever-

al thousands of dollars later she had a real headache. Not only had she not been helped, but her
insurance company refused to pay the doctor's bill.

Sometimes, identifying the agent responsible for
your distress is quite easy—most hay fever sufferers
have a pretty good idea about what causes their seasonal symptoms; others know only too well that they
have to steer clear of touching poison oak or eating
shellfish or fondling cats if they're to stay healthy. At
a guess, perhaps half of those of you who have recurring hypersensitive or classic allergic reactions already
have a good idea about their cause or causes. By a
"good" idea we mean that there is a completely dependable and obvious correlation between being exposed
to an agent and the appearance of your symptoms.
This firm identification of the factor responsible for
your illness—its "etiology" as the doctors label it—is
most likely to apply to conditions (a) having a single
cause and (b) demonstrating an unmistakable link
between exposure and onset of symptoms.

You may not know quite what to do about the
symptoms, but you *definitely* know where they come
from. If you're absolutely sure about the cause of your
problem, you may want to turn to the relevant chapters in Part 4. But if you don't know, or aren't sure,
what is producing your symptoms, or if you're not completely confident of your personal diagnosis, read on.

Whenever the symptoms of an allergic reaction
are slow to develop or are mixed—skin *and* gastric
symptoms occurring as a complex reaction to something that you ate, for instance—finding the specific
agent responsible is always more difficult. One of the

real problems with exposure to allergic or irritant substances is that the body can respond to them in so many different ways. Implausible reactions—in which responses seem to make no sense at all, or seem not to follow any rules—do happen.

> Billy first went on a plane ride when his mother took him from West Palm Beach to Dallas to visit his grandmother. The mother was pleased that the airline had remembered Billy's child's meal, even the candy bar that went with it. Thirty minutes after the meal, however, Billy began to break out in hives. He was in agony; all he could do was scratch frantically at welts that soon covered almost his entire body. His mother couldn't understand it; Billy had never shown this or any other kind of apparent allergic reaction. When they arrived in Dallas, Billy was rushed to an acute care clinic and given an antihistamine. His symptoms quickly disappeared. Ten years later the same thing happened again; everyone attributed the episode to a weird, idiosyncratic reaction. Billy went on to medical school and, during the course of his studies, mentioned his hives to one of his professors. The professor suggested that Billy was allergic to something unusual he ate. After some detective work they found that the trigger was cottonseed oil, which is sometimes used in candy. They learned that Billy had to ingest a substantial amount before any reaction would occur.

To solve a mystery you need to establish means, motive, and opportunity. To determine what is responsible for an irritant or allergic reaction you must answer a chained sequence of questions:

1. Where on your body are your symptoms located?
2. What exactly are your symptoms?
3. Do the symptoms turn up at a particular time of the year? A particular time of the day or week? In a particular place or places?
4. How long do your symptoms ordinarily last?
5. Do your symptoms wake you up—can and do they surface when you are sleeping?
6. What do you do if you fail to come up with a plausible explanation for your symptoms—and what is a plausible explanation?
7. What (if anything) have you done to treat your symptoms?
8. Is there anything that you do that will ease the symptoms or make them go away?

Where Are Your Symptoms Located?

Allergic or hypersensitivity symptoms generally occur either in your airways (nose or lung), skin, or abdomen. Abdominal reactions are virtually always from something you ate. Most reactions to food, if they are allergic, occur within 45 minutes of a meal or snack. In contrast, irritant or infectious reactions in the abdomen may take several hours to develop.

Chuck is a professor of gastroenterology at a large eastern medical school. Several hours after flying east on a business trip, he developed crampy abdominal pain and profuse diarrhea. The only food he had taken was on the plane. He had no trouble recognizing the symptoms of food poisoning, most likely from the rich, whipped-cream-laden dessert that ended the meal.

Some abdominal symptoms are found primarily among those with certain specific ethnic or racial backgrounds.

Joe, an African-American, loved ice cream but it didn't love him. Any time he ate a sundae he became ill. Like millions of other African-Americans, Asians, Jews, and Hispanics, Joe was deficient in an intestinal enzyme known as lactase. This is a harmless deficiency unless you consume something like milk or ice cream that is rich in lactose. In that case the lactose cannot be digested and is converted into gas with considerable bloating and diarrhea. Lactase deficiency grows more pronounced as you become older.

There are other peculiar abdominal reactions that occur with age.

Ira, 58, used to love raw green onions. The trouble is that nowadays he becomes *persona non grata* 45 minutes to an hour after eating them. Like many older adults (men, mainly, in the case of onions) he has lost the ability to digest onions properly and they are converted to smelly methane gas and ammonia. Bran and many other fiber-rich foods have the same effect although, if you eat them regularly, you can partially regain your tolerance for them.

Nasal symptoms are usually easier to diagnose because they turn up almost immediately after exposure when they are allergic in nature. More difficult to pin down is the cause of something called vasomotor rhinitis.

Warren works for the phone company, where his job is to sell Yellow Pages advertising. He is on the road every day and spends most weekday nights in a motel. His nose is always congested and running. He saw several allergists and they were unable to find anything at all other than a chronically congested nose. Of interest, however, was the fact that he always improved when he was at home, especially on long weekends or over vacations. The allergist who finally brought this fact out concluded that the stale motel air, made worse by old, inadequately maintained air conditioners, was responsible for his condition, which is called vasomotor rhinitis.

The most frightening reactions are the ones that affect the lower respiratory system and they, too, occur almost immediately after exposure. These severe, often life-threatening episodes are called anaphylactic reactions and they are discussed in detail in Chapter 14.

Many skin reactions result from direct contact with some irritant or allergen and are collectively called contact dermatitis.

Sally found that earrings made her ear lobes swell and become very painful. Her dermatologist soon determined that she was sensitive to the nickel used in inexpensive jewelry. When she started wearing nickel-free (and much more expensive) pieces, the problem went away.

Skin sensitivity reactions can be quite severe and often require only the slightest exposure to appear.

Matt, exquisitely susceptible to poison ivy, scrupulously avoided contact with the plant. Even so, he seemed to have an outbreak several times a year and his mother couldn't figure out why. It turned out that Matt's dog was coming into contact with the plant and when Matt petted the dog he also rubbed onto his hands minute quantities of the oily poison-ivy irritant clinging to the dog's fur—and that was enough to trigger the symptoms.

What Exactly Are Your Symptoms?

Allergic or toxic reactions usually are expressed as symptoms that affect one or more of the four major bodily systems (*see* Table 8). Now look at Figure 1 (p. 53). It represents the various bodily sites in which the more common allergic or toxic reactions may be expressed. You will see that any one cause is capable of involving one or more of the systems; the cause, whatever it is, may express itself as cutaneous (3) symptoms alone, or it may produce symptoms in any two (3, 4, cutaneous and gastric, for example), three (1, 3, 4), or even all four systems. Since you probably know your symptoms all too well, follow the prompts in the box in Figure 1 to launch your quest for their cause or causes. Depending on your symptoms, Figure 1 will refer you to one or more of a number of decision charts or algorithms—Figures 2 through 5—that will lead you through a step-by-step sequence of questions; at the end of the sequence you should be pointed toward a possible cause or causes. (In doing this, take note that the decision charts try to answer the vital questions listed earlier.)

Table 8
Bodily Systems Affected by Allergic or Irritant Reactions*

System affected	Specific location	Most common symptoms
Upper respiratory	Nose, sinuses (often with involvement of eyes, ears, palate)	Frequent sneezing, runny nose, teary eyes, itchy ears and palate
Lower respiratory	Major airways, lungs, chest	Shortness of breath, wheezing, coughing, tightness in chest
Cutaneous (skin)	Anywhere on the body	Inflammation, itching, rashes, sores, blisters or other skin eruptions
Gastric	Stomach or intestine	Abdominal pain, nausea, vomiting, diarrhea, feelings of overfulness, discomfort

*Other reactions of bodily systems or symptoms *possibly* triggered by allergens or toxins include fatigue, headache, apathy, sleeplessness, constipation, dysuria.

What to Do If You Fail to Come up with a Plausible Explanation for Your Symptoms

If you cannot account for or attach a reasonable cause to your symptoms on your own, and if the symptoms are troublesome, then you need to look into your plight more deeply. To do this you may need help. Chapter 17 catalogs resources that may be available and useful to you. At this stage it may be appropriate to remind you that, as with most other problems in

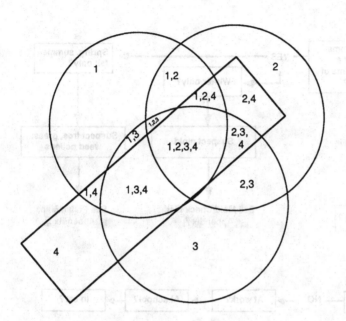

Symptom(s)		Consult Figure(s)
1	Upper Respiratory (UR)	2
2	Lower Respiratory (LR)	3
3	Cutaneous (C)	4
4	Gastric (G)	5
1&2	UR & LR	2 & 3
1&3	UR & C	2 & 4
1&4	UR & G	2 & 5
2&3	LR & C	3 & 4
2&4	LR & G	4 & 5
3&4	C & G	4 & 5
1&2&3	UR & LR & C	2 & 3 & 4
1&2&4	UR & LR & G	2 & 4 & 5
2&3&4	LR & C & G	3 & 4 & 5
1&2&3&4	UR & LR & C & G	see pages
		54 to 59

Figure 1.

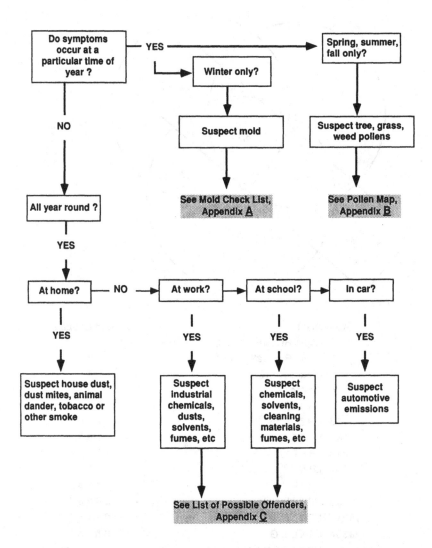

Figure 2. Common causes of allergen or irritant triggered upper respiratory symptoms.

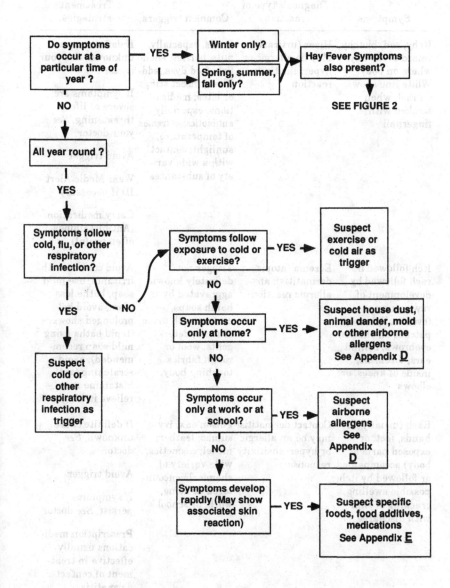

Figure 3. Common causes of allergen or irritant triggered lower respiratory symptoms.

Symptoms	Diagnosis/type of reaction	Common triggers	Treatment strategies
Itchy, red, blotchy, raised areas anywhere on body. White line shows on rash when stroked with fingernail	Hives (urticaria). May be allergic or hypersensitivity reaction	Foods, especially nuts, berries, shellfish; food dyes, additives; insect stings or bites; medications, especially antibiotics; extremes of temperature, sunlight; contact with a wide variety of substances	If definite cause unknown, *See* your doctor

If symptoms are severe or life-threatening, *See* your doctor

Avoid trigger

Wear Medic-Alert ID if necessary

Carry medication. (Antihistamines often useful) |
| Itch followed by rash followed by development of raw, runny or (eventually) scaly patches on cheeks, eyebrows, behind ears, forearms, inside of knees, or elbows | Eczema (atopic dermatitis); an allergic reaction | Trigger not definitely known; aggravated by harsh soaps, contact with urine or feces, detergents, wool or rough fabrics touching body. | Avoid contact with irritants, use mild soap, bathe less often, avoid hot prolonged showers (tepid baths using mild soap recommended); avoid scratching (antihistamine may relieve itching) |
| Rash (usually on hands, feet, or exposed parts of body) accompanied or followed by itch, possible swelling, cracking of skin with discharge | Contact dermatitis/ may be an allergic or hypersensitivity response | Poison oak, ivy sumac; leather; nickel; cosmetics; wide variety of chemicals encountered at home, work, or school. | If definite cause unknown, *See* doctor

Avoid trigger

If symptoms persist, *See* doctor

Prescription medications usually effective in treatment of contact dermatitis |

Figure 4. Symptoms, diagnosis, triggers, and treatment. strategies for various skin allergies or irritants

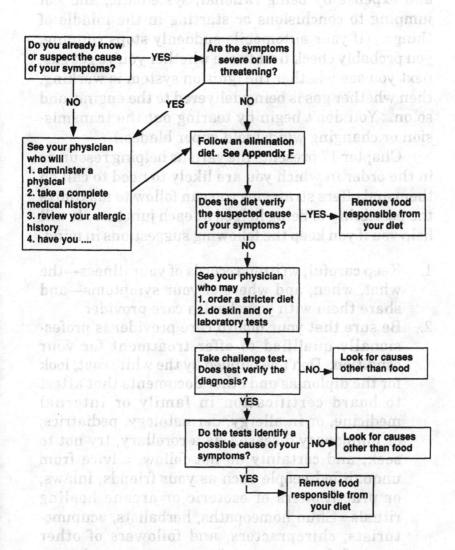

Figure 5. Finding the cause of food allergy or intolerance.

life, you can save yourself a lost of needless trouble
and expense by being rational, systematic, and not
jumping to conclusions or starting in the middle of
things. (If your automobile suddenly stops running,
you probably check first to see whether you've got gas;
next you see whether the ignition system is working,
then whether gas is being delivered to the engine, and
so on. You don't begin by tearing out the transmis-
sion or changing windshield wiper blades.)

Chapter 17 presents the various helping resources
in the order in which you are likely to need to call on
them and offers strategies you can follow to maximize
the possibility of being helped at each juncture. It will
help you if you keep the following suggestions in mind.

1.   Keep careful, written records of your illness—the
     what, when, and where of your symptoms—and
     share them with your health care provider.
2.   Be sure that your health care provider is profes-
     sionally qualified to offer treatment for your
     condition. Don't be blinded by the white coat; look
     for the diplomas and other documents that attest
     to board certification in family or internal
     medicine, or in allergy, dermatology, pediatrics,
     or pulmonary disease. As a corollary, try not to
     seek, and certainly do not follow, advice from
     unqualified people such as your friends, inlaws,
     or practitioners of esoteric or arcane healing
     rituals. Shun homeopaths, herbalists, acupunc-
     turists, chiropractors, and followers of other
     crank, fad, or unproven treatment approaches, or
     ones that are irrelevant to your condition.
3.   If you are prescribed medication, it must be for
     something. *Insist* on knowing what the medicine

is being prescribed for, what it is, what its effect will be, what side effects it may cause, and what you should do if one occurs. And, you must take the medication strictly according to directions.
4. Do not be reluctant or hesitant to seek a second opinion, or a referral, if the treatment does not seem to be succeeding.
5. When the cause of your condition is finally determined—and this may require an elaborate and prolonged series of tests—conscientiously avoid it. See Chapter 5 and the relevant chapters in Part 5 to develop appropriate avoidance tactics.

What Can Be Done to Treat Your Symptoms?

If the cause of your condition is unavoidable, the question of how to treat the inevitable symptoms comes up. For some reactions—asthma and hay fever in particular—there are medications available that, when properly used, can effectively prevent the appearance or control the severity of symptoms. In the case of mild, occasional episodes of these allergic conditions, there are even over-the-counter (OTC) medications that can greatly reduce the intensity of an episode. Mild, seasonal or chronic hay fever can be helped by OTC antihistamines; moderate to severe attacks can be ameliorated or avoided by using antihistamines or intranasal steroids. Mild asthma attacks can be eased by appropriate use of OTC inhalers; more serious symptoms can be managed by use of prescription inhalers, theophylline, cromolyn sodium, or steroids.

Skin and gastric problems are somewhat more difficult to treat and we cannot stress too firmly the risks involved in self-medication. Oftentimes skin irritations are made worse by either applying OTC salves or ointments that intensify or spread the rash, or by using cosmetic coverups that also have the effect of worsening the symptoms. With chronic skin problems you will be better off seeking and following professional medical advice.

Problems that result from gastric allergies or irritant reactions are best treated by avoiding altogether the foodstuff or food additive that provokes the symptoms. There isn't much you or anyone else can do to relieve the symptoms; they have to run their course. However, when the material ingested also provokes skin (hives), vascular (headaches, dizziness), or respiratory (wheezing and shortness of breath) problems, there are medications you can take to relieve the discomfort. Talk to your doctor to get recommendations about appropriate medication and prescriptions, if needed. One word of warning, though. When something you eat or drink does trigger hives, breathing difficulties, or a drop in blood pressure, this is a serious and potentially dangerous complication and you should definitely have medical advice on the appropriate countermeasures to take, should carry medication for use in an emergency, and should wear identification that will let others know of your problem, and what measures will rescue you from your emergency.

What You Can Do to Ease or Prevent Symptoms

People often ask if there is anything they can do—lifestyle changes they can make, for example—that will make their symptoms less severe or vanish altogether.

We have already indicated that a carefully worked out and followed avoidance strategy can go a long way toward preventing allergic or hypersensitive episodes. Much of this book aims at providing you with knowledge and skills to do just that.

Beyond avoidance, there are other things you can do to make your life easier and more comfortable. If you know when or under what conditions your symptoms are likely to occur you can, with some complaints like seasonal hay fever, initiate a preventive course of medication before the sneezing and sniffling is due to start.

With asthma, you have at least a couple of steps you can take to ward off or dull the severity of an episode. Breathing and drainage exercises done regularly (and accompanied by a systematic and diligent effort to keep in good physical condition) can help to cut down the severity of attacks markedly. In addition, an impending attack of asthma is ordinarily preceded by a fall-off in lung capacity. Lung capacity can easily be measured by using a peak-flow meter, a simple and inexpensive device. If these measurements are taken and recorded regularly—twice daily, morning and evening—it is quite possible to forecast when an asthma attack is on the way and to take medications that anticipate its arrival and reduce its severity.

Apart from these steps, there is one additional precaution you can take. People do not like to feel vulnerable to or at the mercy of substances that can't be seen at all or, if they can, look perfectly innocuous, and don't affect other people the way that they do you.

Thus, if there have been no symptoms for a period of time, there is the temptation to check and see whether the sensitivity is history. So, you sample just a little bit of whatever it is that upsets your stomach, or you decide to use a forbidden cosmetic to hide a skin problem, or you stage an encounter just to see whether dust mites still carry their old power.

This wish to be well and whole is endearingly human, but sensitivities or allergies do not go away. Even asthma, whose attacks tend to become less severe with age, can recur at any time. Don't push your luck.

Points to Remember

Identifying the exact cause of your allergy or hypersensitivity is the key to managing or controlling your symptoms. This chapter tells you how to go about this process of detection systematically and rationally.

In our experience most people have a good idea about what triggers their problem; when it is not definitely known, carefully assembling and assessing data from a variety of sources should unmask the culprit. Simple things like the nature and site of the symptoms, where you are or the time of day or the season of the year that they appear, can point to a specific cause or significantly narrow the list of suspects. Once the field is cut down, tests are available that can generally pinpoint the agent.

Detecting the allergen or irritant responsible for your condition is crucial because the most effective countermeasure available to you is simply to avoid the trigger. Though medications allow treatment of some symptoms, we believe that it is infinitely preferable to know and stay well away from the cause of your difficulties. Drugs can be helpful some of the time, but you will be better off, physically, psychologically, and economically if you can build a lifestyle that makes them unnecessary.

CHAPTER 5

Strategies for Avoiding Causes of Allergic or Irritant Reactions

By following the procedures we have spelled out in Chapter 4 you should now have gained a precise idea of whatever it is that triggers your allergic or irritant reaction.

The next and most important step toward competent management of your symptoms is to develop strategies for avoiding the cause of your difficulty. Part V, Chapters 10–16, outlines steps you can take to escape the allergens or irritants you encounter in your various milieus—at home, work, school, and so on. These specific suggestions grow out of a set of basic principles that, if followed scrupulously, should enable you to anticipate and avoid the source of your troubles.

We prefer this "proactive" approach; when it comes to allergies, avoiding causes (and, thus, the symptoms they provoke) is infinitely preferable, on all counts, to simply reacting and treating the symptoms once they are established in your body.

In a sense the process you will follow resembles that of a skillful driver who religiously monitors the actions of other drivers, works out a continually unfolding plan designed to keep risk to a minimum, adjusts his or her behavior to conditions, and has an emergency plan ready in the event that other mea-

sures break down. We call these personal qualities—
the heart of an effective avoidance plan—vigilance,
defensiveness, adaptability, and resourcefulness.

Vigilance

Vigilance requires that you know the sources of
your discomfort with absolute clarity and then take
whatever steps are necessary to keep out of their way.

June is extremely sensitive to milk and milk products. At home her diet scrupulously excludes milk
and other foods containing milk, including such
unlikely vehicles as dry salami or frankfurters.
She reads food container labels down to the last
word and she knows all of the various disguises
that milk can assume, lactose being the main one.
When she dines out at a restaurant she selects
carefully and when she is not sure about an item
on the menu she asks exactly what it contains
and how it is prepared. If the information cannot
be supplied she goes on to another choice. She is
also likely to say how something is to be cooked.
(No sautéing in butter or margarine, for example,
because some margarines contain milk.) At the
home of friends she takes pains to let her hosts
know ahead of time about her problem so that
they can be guided appropriately. Finally, she
never eats anything she is unsure about. By taking these unfailing precautions, going on three
years now, June has managed to avoid the violent gastric symptoms that once plagued her.

"The condition upon which God hath given liberty to man is eternal vigilance..." One problem you
will have to be prepared to live with is that eternal

vigilance may stigmatize you as a crank or a nuisance. Other people will notice and wonder and perhaps comment critically about your efforts to safeguard yourself. But your allergies, your reactions to irritants, will cause you much more suffering if you let your vigilance flag.

Another problem with vigilance is that it isn't easy. You have to do some serious studying, you have to organize information and develop a plan, you need to work on it full-time, and you can't afford any slip-ups. If you're allergic to dust mites, we tell you in Chapter 12 how to eradicate these pests; the management process is meticulous and tedious; housecleaning at any level is a drag and dust mite housecleaning is a world-class drag. You may find yourself saying that the cleaning can slide for a few days, that everything looks OK, that it'll do. Maybe so. And then again, maybe not. Probably the latter. Vigilance is the smaller discomfort.

Defensiveness

In one sense a defensive posture is a selfish one; you assume it to minimize the possibility of harm to yourself. Wearing your seat belt, sticking to the speed limit, maintaining a prudent distance from the car in front of you, letting other drivers know of your intentions, all of these defensive moves ultimately aim at keeping you safe.

Being constantly on the defensive is difficult, boring, and frustrating—whether you're talking about automobiles or allergens. And, defensiveness only promotes safety, without ensuring it, so that there is al-

ways the temptation to take a chance. When it comes
to allergens or irritants, here are some of the tempta-
tions you will encounter and will need to spurn.

The Temptation to Test the Limits

Allergies and hypersensitivity reactions are a lifelong condition. Some symptoms may at times remit—
for instance, asthma ordinarily becomes less severe
in children as they grow older and their airways en-
large. However, the vulnerability to the disease is still
there and it can recur at any time when the conditions are "right." However, where symptoms have
been absent for a time, there is a strong tendency to
think of oneself as being "cured" and to test this hypothesis by directly confronting and experiencing the
known cause.

> As a child Margaret had severe attacks of hives
> with associated breathing difficulties when
> she ate strawberries. After her third episode
> Margaret's mother implanted firmly in her the
> idea that eating strawberries was bad for her and
> would certainly bring on the "strawberry rash."
> Margaret went through her later childhood, ado-
> lescence, and young adulthood without ever eat-
> ing another strawberry. Then, when she was in
> her late twenties she began wondering if she'd
> outgrown her sensitivity and was missing some-
> thing good in her life. She decided to give the fruit
> another try. The rash developed immediately,
> serious breathing difficulties followed, and Mar-
> garet had to be taken to the emergency room and
> treated before the symptoms cleared. Mother
> knew best in Margaret's case.

The lesson here is not to play games with your condition; accept it, take whatever steps are necessary to keep it from recurring, and stick with them.

The Desire to Make "Nice-Nice"

Social pressures can push you into situations in which you let down your guard. Friends or relatives can urge or force you to do things that, deep down, you know may be harmful. "Aw, come on. Try a glass of this modest little self-effacing Pinot Noir. A tiny hit won't hurt a big girl like you," the argument might go and, rather than cause hurt to the hostess or take the abuse that would follow refusal, you go along knowing full well that the sulfites in the wine will have you struggling for breath. If you know that what you're being urged to do will be bad for you, either decline the invitation or offer as gracefully as you can (or, as bluntly as you need to) or, if you see absolutely no way of declining, accept the glass. Just don't touch the contents. Leave them, spill them on the damask tablecloth, pour them into the philodendron, whatever. Just don't drink them.

The Tendency to Keep Mum About Your Condition

Many people don't like to admit to a health problem because they see (and believe others see in such admissions) a sign of weakness or inadequacy. They prefer either to conceal the condition by acting as if it doesn't exist or by trying to overcome it. Though most allergies can be treated with appropriate medications or even moderated with lifestyle changes, the potential to react to triggers is original factory equipment.

Your misdeeds, whatever they are, are not likely to have caused or intensified your allergy or hypersensitivity, so no shame or blame should attach to you, and you should not be in the least hesitant to tell others that tobacco smoke makes you wheeze or their cat makes you sneeze.

Suffering silently is closely linked to another common disposition—the outright denial of the existence of a condition. In part this tendency traces back to the once predominant idea that allergic or sensitivity reactions (asthma in particular) were attributable to psychological causes. The hypothesis that allergic diseases are psychogenic in origin has been thoroughly discredited, but the idea still persists, even among some physicians who, of all people, ought to know better. Thus, many individuals, victims of this myth, either deny outright or minimize the existence of their very real symptoms, believing deep down that wheezing is but prelude to the entry of the men in the white coats.

Allergic or hypersensitive reactions are real. They arise from explicit physical causes, they are uncomfortable, and, in many instances, dangerous to the point of being life-threatening. You need to accept them as part of the fabric of your life, and you need to develop and employ strategies that defend you from their causes and enable you to acknowledge them fully and openly.

Adaptability

You cannot adapt to an allergen or irritant; you can adapt to the conditions that interdict the causative agent, making it difficult for the agent to affect you adversely. The kind of process we are talking about here is one that enables you to make behavioral changes, changes in your habits and style of living that allow you to pursue a more complete, comfortable, satisfying, fuller round of life activities.

Successful avoidance of antigens will require you to change at least some of your activities: you may have to give up pleasant things, such as the glass of wine with dinner, the occasional pepperoni pizza, or smoking; it may cut out satisfying activities like certain forms of exercise, driving in a convertible with the top down, long hot showers; it may confine you to certain areas of your home some or much of the time; it may rule out the pleasure of keeping a pet; it may impose regimens of environmental cleanliness or personal care on you that are onerous and tedious; it may make aspects of grooming, beautification, or personal adornment impossible; it may force you, at home, work, or in school, to wear uncomfortable and conspicuous protective gear some of the time; it may curtail how much and by what means you travel; it may force you to make changes in your occupation.

Adaptability is nothing more than having the willingness, the resolve, and the internal resources to make those adjustments that your condition, whatever it is, demands. Making such changes may be absurdly simple.

Each spring Matthew had severe hay fever triggered by tree pollens. He installed an air conditioning unit with high efficiency filters in his bedroom, removed the pollen-catching decor, and sealed the room off from the out-of-doors and the

rest of the house by weatherstripping doors and
windows tightly. During the height of the brief
pollen season, he spent most of his at home time
in the bedroom and suffered almost no discomfort.

On the other hand, your allergies may require profound changes that dictate the curtailment of some
activities, a change of occupation, or other major adjustments. Overcoming ingrained patterns or habits
of behavior is seldom easy, even though the illness
may provide a seemingly compelling incentive to
change. Fortunately, help in effecting behavioral
change can be found. Various sources and modes of
assistance are listed in Chapter 17.

Resourcefulness

"The hedgehog knows one thing; the fox knows
many things." To succeed in avoiding the triggers of
your allergies you need to know many things—you
need to be resourceful.

Intelligent and imaginative use of your resources
is the final principle on which effective avoidance of
allergens or irritants rests. There are several guide-
lines that, if they are followed, will help keep you from
wasting time, energy, and money as you strive to eliminate the source of your problem.

Be absolutely certain that you have hard evidence—in the form of incontrovertible observational
data or the results of standard medical tests—of the
cause of your allergic reaction. The readiness of people
to accept unsubstantiated, off-the-cuff opinions from
others who have no qualifications whatsoever to make
such judgments about the causes of allergy problems

continues to astonish and appall us. Check and verify
the training and experience of your health care provider before accepting a diagnosis; do not hesitate to
get a second opinion if you have any doubts whatsoever about the verdict you have been handed.

This questioning attitude will also serve you well
as you develop procedures for avoiding your trigger.
For example, if you have pollen-caused hay fever, you
will probably want to think about getting some sort of
device that will cleanse and purify the air in all or
part of your home. Before making any move to acquire
a unit, look into Chapter 12 where the specifications
for and features of various types of air conditioners
are spelled out. Figure out the type and size of unit
that you will require and then try to rent the desired
model from a medical supply house or other purveyor
for a trial period before consummating the sale. At
the same time, insure that the conditions under which
it operates are such that it can work effectively; if you
set up an air cleaner in a space that is not effectively
sealed from the invasion of pollen through doors, windows, return air registers, and the like, no unit will
be of much help to you. As a general rule you can
trust the declarations about the unit's technical specifications, which ordinarily accompany or are stamped
on the product, but be especially wary of the manufacturer's or distributor's claims for efficacy; these tend
to be inflated and based on dubious testimonials.

Resourcefulness depends on securing and being
willing and able to weigh information. One useful
source of information is this book, and the helpful
Appendixes that make up its final section. Your family physician, allergist, or dermatologist can also help

you greatly, especially if you insist (as is your right) that the information and instructions you receive are delivered in terms that you fully understand.

Reference libraries (and librarians), especially those in universities, teaching hospitals, or medical schools can also help you to dig out information you will need to make informed choices.

Another aspect of resourcefulness is the readiness to admit that a stratagem is not working and to begin to think of alternative approaches. All too often people get locked into ineffective treatment modes and follow them slavishly—sometimes for years—fueled by the hope that things will eventually improve. Allergies and hypersensitivities usually respond with gratifying swiftness to removal of the triggering agent; if your symptoms don't begin to let up within a week or two after the avoidance procedure is put in place, either you are not following the procedure closely enough, or it is not appropriate, or the cause has been misidentified.

Points to Remember

In sum, the specific measures you take to avoid whatever is responsible for your allergy or hypersensitivity depends on the nature of the reaction, the agent causing it, and where it occurs—home, work, school, etc. Specific avoidance steps are spelled out in Part V, and the Appendix provides additional information that will help you to develop effective strategies to get rid of your problem. Whether or not your plan of action works really depends on you and your ability to devise, install, and follow the course of action appro-

priate to your condition. Successfully evicting allergens or irritants from your life ultimately depends on
having and exercising the personal qualities that make
it possible for you to be unfailingly vigilant, defensive, or self-protective, adaptable, and resourceful.
Avoidance techniques—your best tactics—will not
work unless you make every effort to see that they
work. Though blaming the doctor for the lack of suc-
cess of your treatment is a more or less ritual exercise, probably a majority of failures in allergy treatment are attributable to the allergic person's inability or unwillingness to follow the steps that were laid
out to manage the problem, or their simple disregard
or neglect. Be warned, though: those efforts may place
considerable physical, psychological, and social bur-
dens on you and your family. The costs and sacrifices
can be high, but the benefits, as measured in improved
health and well-being, and in heightened self-esteem,
easily outweigh them.

PART 4

CARRIERS OF ALLERGENS AND IRRITANTS

CHAPTER 6

The Food You Eat

Composition—The Principal Food Offenders
and the Problems They Cause;
Additives and Contaminents

Food wrongly catches the blame for many of the allergy-like reactions we suffer. There are a couple of reasons for this misattribution. First, most reactions to food are not truly allergic; rather, they are irritant in character. Second, where the reaction is allergic, it is considerably more likely to be caused by some additive or contaminant found in the food rather than the food itself.

Jill has had headaches all of her life. During her required health class in college, the instructor had mentioned a disease called cerebral allergy. According to the instructor, some headaches result from an allergic reaction to something eaten. Jill read everything she could find on the topic, but she was no fool and it soon became apparent that few reputable scientists believed that headaches were the result of an allergy. She did find out, however, that many foods contain chemicals called vasoactive amines that can cause headaches in some people. Jill made a list of these foods and removed them from her diet—ripe cheese, bananas, and anchovies among many others. When she did this her headaches did not stop entirely, but they occurred less often and were less severe.

Allergic Versus Hypersensitive Reactions to Food

A truly allergic reaction, as we pointed out in Chapter 1, occurs when a foreign substance enters the body and triggers the production of Immunoglobulin E (IgE) which, in its turn, sets off a complex chain of events that end with the release of histamine. The histamine provokes allergic symptoms—respiratory difficulties, skin disorders, GI troubles. Only a few foods are known to be capable of causing this allergic sequence in susceptible individuals, and only a small percentage of all individuals are likely to be so affected. This is not to dispute the fact that some foods disagree with some people. Most of us steer clear of a food or two because we know that if we eat it we'll live to regret it. But, in most instances, incompatibility with certain foods is not an allergic reaction. Rather, the food, whatever it is, triggers your reaction directly without involving the immune mechanisms in your body. Knowing whether your reaction to a food is allergic or hypersensitive in origin is important. Important, too, is knowing exactly what it is that causes your symptoms. Although allergic or irritant symptoms may be indistinguishable from one another—diarrhea, after all, is diarrhea and hives are hives—what you do about your symptoms depends crucially on whether or not they are allergic. In either case, you will doubtless work to avoid exposure to whatever provokes your symptoms. If your reaction is an irritant one, avoidance of the offending substance is your only option. Allergies can be controlled medically by antihistamines or other anti-allergic response drugs; reactions to irritants cannot be so readily controlled.

> There is a little Mom and Pop bakery in a town not far from where one of the authors lives. The bakery turns out an exemplary apple fritter—light, crisp, utterly delicious. Whenever he passes through that town the author stops in at the bakery, buys, and eats one of those fritters in the full knowledge that he will inevitably have a modest case of indigestion the rest of the day.

Though the author willingly pays the price for his minor act of self-indulgence, other hypersensitive or allergic reactions can be much more severe—even life-threatening in some instances—and scrupulous avoidance of the known trigger offers the best recourse and, with an irritant, the only one.

> Cheryl knows very well how allergic she is to nuts. She once nearly died when she went into shock after eating a breakfast bar that contained walnuts. Nuts are a common cause of food allergy and those who are allergic to them must be careful to the point of being phobic in avoiding them.

To help you decide whether your symptoms are truly allergic or a response to an irritant, refer to Tables 9 and 10. Table 9 tells the ways in which antibodies can trigger symptoms; Table 10 lists the many reactions to food that occur whose mechanisms are unknown and probably do not add up to a true allergy in the medical sense. The number of people whose complaints appear in Table 10 probably outnumber those

Table 9
Substances Released by IgE
That Trigger Allergic Symptoms

Substance released	Symptoms triggered
Histamine	Itching, swelling, wheezing, runny nose
Serotonin	Swelling,[1] coughing
Prostaglandins	Swelling, cough, wheezing, abdominal pain
Platelet activating factor	Wheezing

[1]Swelling refers to edema; it can occur almost anywhere including face, arms, neck and legs.

Table 10
Non-Allergic (Irritant or Intolerant) Reactions to Foods

Food	Reaction
Dairy products	Bloating, diarrhea, rashes
Cheese, sausage, wine, etc.	Headaches
Wine	Wheezing
Eggs	Rashes
Tomatoes	Rashes, abdominal pain
Citrus fruits	Mouth ulcers, diarrhea
Grains	Diarrhea, bloating
Onions	Gas, flatulence
MSG[1]	Headache

[1]MSG (monosodium glutamate) is included in this table because it has (sadly!) become such a common food additive.

who fall in Table 9 by at least one thousand to one. Foods do have the potential for making you sick in a variety of ways, but the odds are that the sickness is not allergic; you simply have an intolerance.

Foods—and the Stuff We Eat

What we eat is not simple, pure unadulterated food. Vegetables are helped in the growth cycle by pesticides, herbicides, and fungicides—all of which persist as residues. When processed after picking, they receive chemical additives that preserve, color, or otherwise enhance their appearance or taste or are thought to carry health bonuses—vitamins, trace elements, minerals. Animals, the source of meats, milk, and eggs, are routinely dosed with hormones and antibiotics to spur growth and ward off disease; these additives find their way to your table and your stomach. Even fish and shellfish are not free of chemicals and other reaction-causing substances.

There are, altogether, several hundred chemicals that are routinely added to food. Almost none of them has been tested for safety and their effects on humans have not been assessed for consumer health and safety. Those responsible suppliers who actually make the effort to test some of their products for insecticide or herbicide residues do not have the capability to look for all possible contaminants and, even if they could, have no dependable information on their potential effects. (For an extended discussion of this point, see Chapter 10.)

In addition to additives and residues, there are contaminants that may accidentally get into or can-

Table 11
Common Food Additives and Contaminants
That May Produce Allergic or Irritant Reactions

A. Additives
1. Sulfur dioxide
2. Benzoate
3. Tartrazine
4. Chelating agents, e.g., EDTA
5. Sulfites
6. MSG (monosodium glutamate)
7. Food dyes (hundreds of them!!!)

B. Contaminants
1. Insect parts
2. Rodent parts
3. Rodent excrement
4. Antibiotics
5. Hormones
6. Bacteria
7. Mold
8. Parasites
9. Hepatitis virus

not be kept from food as it is processed. Insect parts and animal matter are a regular (below certain arbitrary US Food and Drug Administration determined levels), and a permissible part of your diet. Microorganisms such as salmonella occasionally invade and flourish in processed foods. Indeed, much of what passes as "stomach flu" is more likely to be caused by a bacterial infection.

Spills or accidents during processing can introduce almost anything into food products—fuels, solvents, cleansing agents, and so on. Any one of them, in sufficient dosage, is capable of making you sick; a few of them also can provoke allergic or sensitivity symptoms.

We have identified some common residues, additives, and contaminants known to cause allergic or hypersensitivity reactions, and these are listed in Table 11; Appendix E names the more important foods known to cause the same type of allergic or hypersensitivity reactions.

Food producers and processors advance a number of arguments to justify the wholesale and largely irresponsible introduction of chemicals into foodstuffs. They say that they are responding to public demand (as if advertising were not a device to create demand) by reducing costs, cutting waste, and improving the appearance of their products.

Yet, the consumer is never consulted when the decision is made to add substances like tartrazine or sulfiting agents to foods; these chemicals simply prolong product shelf life, "improve" appearance, and, not coincidentally, boost profits. They have no food value. And, if you get sick from these potent irritants that's your—or your insurance company's—problem. The food merchants don't pick up the medical bills when their products make you sick.

We point out in Chapter 10 that we do not give carte blanche to so-called "health" foods. We view claims that a given product is "natural" or "organic" as either meaningless or subject to considerable skepticism and the extravagant claims about the health values of most "health" foods have not been backed by credible scientific evidence. Yet, the food merchants are right. If you and others like you learn to read package labels carefully and conscientiously, and if you then refuse to buy the overpriced "chemical banquets" they serve up (and a lax government permits them to vend), the manufacturers may get the message and put a stop to their heedless, harmful, and, in the final analysis, greed-fueled practices.

How to Read a Package Label

Package labeling is a hit and miss proposition. Fresh foods (meat and produce) are not required to have labels, even though they have doubtless seen a number of chemicals somewhere along the line.

Canned, packaged, processed, or frozen foods do list what is in the package—seemingly—and in their order of importance. It pays to remember, though, that a simple declaration "Ingredients: Broccoli" on a package of frozen broccoli says nothing about what was on the broccoli when it arrived at the processing plant. The same thing is true of any canned, packaged, or processed food. The implication on the label is that the principal food ingredients that went into the product were "pure" or "natural." If you believe that you won't have any trouble accepting the Tooth Fairy. So, the first rule in label reading is to be skeptical. The second rule is to read the label carefully to see whether the foodstuff contains whatever it is that causes you trouble. It makes sense to do this in the store, before buying. Plan your shopping trips to allow you the time to do this. And always check—even if you are buying a product that has been safe for you in the past. Ingredients can and do change all the time, and you can be sure that you won't get a warning when it happens. Here is a list of ingredients taken from a loaf of Wheat French Bread. The items superscripted[1] are known to cause allergic reactions in susceptible persons; those superscripted[2] are also known to provoke hypersensitivity reactions. The items written in italics probably make no contribution whatsoever to what is otherwise a healthy diet and need not have been added to what is a staple food.

Wheat French Bread

Enriched flour[2] (wheat flour, malted barley flour, *niacin, reduced iron, thiamine mononitrate, riboflavin,* water, whole wheat flour[1,2], yeast,[1,2] high fructose corn syrup,[2] molasses,[2] salt, partially hydrogenated vegetable oils, soybean[1,2] and/or cottonseed,[1,2] oil, wheat bran,[2] egg whites,[2] cracked wheat,[2] rye meal,[2] *gluten,*[2] *caramel color,* corn flour,[2] honey, soy grits,[1,2] *calcium sulfate, monocalcium phosphate, diacetyl tartaric acid ester of diglycerides, mono and diglycerides, food starch–modified, sodium stearyl lactylate,*[2] *ammonium sulfate, fungal enzymes,*[1,2] *ascorbic acid, potassium bromate, potassium iodate.*

Had enough?

Foods Causing Allergic or Irritant Sensitivity Reactions

Although there is probably someone, somewhere, who is sensitive or allergic to any food you might name, there are only a few categories of foodstuffs that are likely to provoke reactions in significant numbers of individuals. These foods in adults are: grains, nuts, fruits, and meats. In children they commonly include milk and eggs.

Grain

The grains or cereals that we consume include wheat, oat, corn, rye, and rice. These are the main ingredients of breads, cakes, pastries, and pasta, and they also serve as fillers in many processed foods. Any of them can trigger allergic reactions, although rice is only rarely an offender. For the other grains, the most common manifestations of sensitivity or intolerance are expressed as abdominal complaints like bloating, diarrhea, or constipation. Flatulence almost always accompanies food sensitivity and represents a special problem for older people. Flatulence also shows up in people who consume the brans that many people take because it is believed by some (and so claimed enthusiastically and extravagantly by cereal producers) that bran lowers cholesterol. The bran is not readily digested by the enzymes in your intestines. Instead it is broken down by the bacteria that live in your gut. These bacteria, instead of digesting bran, destroy it and as a product of the resulting chemical reaction, release methane gas. The result? Embarrassment at the least.

Less serious sensitivity reactions to grains, like reactions to any food, are not easy to pin down to a specific cause. Although traditional allergy skin testing or RAST testing may be helpful, for the most part they are not recommended. First, they can be dangerous, eliciting severe reactions; second, they are imprecise so that a negative test result does not necessarily rule out intolerance, nor a positive one confirm

Table 12
Clinical Features of Gluten Enteropathy

1. Diarrhea
2. Abdominal pain
3. Aches in joints
4. Floating stools (steatorrhea)
5. Weight loss
6. Family history of similar disease

it. One of the reasons for this difficulty is that it may not only be, for example, corn that you are reacting to. You may be reacting to the way the corn has been prepared or processed. Corn on the cob, fresh from your garden, is not the same as corn that has been harvested, cooked, packaged, canned, frozen, and/or mixed with any of a number of other foods and bombarded with chemicals.

A more serious type of reaction to grains is a condition called celiac sprue, or gluten enteropathy. People with sprue cannot tolerate gluten, a protein found in wheat. They react violently to wheat and wheat products, developing severe diarrhea, weight loss, and fatigue. Most people with gluten sensitivity are of Northern European ancestry. Early diagnosis is a must if severe wasting is not to occur. The features of gluten enteropathy are sketched in Table 12.

Nuts

Nuts rate a separate listing because, among all the foods, reactions to nuts represent the most serious ones—incredibly swift and, in some instances, potentially lethal. In fact, true allergy to nuts is not uncommon and may be caused by any of the ordinary

Table 13
Common Foods That Contain Nuts

1. Cereals
2. Breakfast bars
3. Many fast ("nutritional") foods, e.g., granola bars, fiber bars
4. Candy bars
5. Some cooking oils
6. Peanut butter, peanut crunch, etc.
7. Cakes, cookies, some flavors of ice cream
8. Many types of "grain" breads

varieties—walnuts, cashews, hazel nuts, macadamia, pecans, Brazil nuts, almonds, and so on. Nuts are widely used in breakfast bars and all sorts of other processed "instant energy" foods; if you react to nuts, be sure the product has a proper label and that you read it carefully before eating. Foods that are made with, or frequently contain, nuts are named in Table 13.

You will note that we have not mentioned peanuts along with the nuts. That is because peanuts are not a nut; rather they are a legume, members of the pea family. However, when it comes to causing reactions, peanuts are often to blame, and if you react to peanuts, check labels not only for peanuts in any form, but also for peanut oil, which is sometimes used in food preparation. For this reason we are including peanuts in Table 13.

Fruit

Fruit reactions may be the most difficult to nail down, simply because so many reactions to fruit are

Table 14
Typical Allergic or Irritant
Reactions to Fruits

1. Rashes
2. Hives
3. Bloating, flatulence
4. Diarrhea
5. Abdominal pain
6. Cold sores

possible. Table 14 catalogs the various reactions that can occur to fruits. Citrus fruits (oranges, grapefruit, tangerines, lemons) are generally the worst offenders, especially in children. Reactions to citrus are usually easy to spot because the temporal relationship between ingestion and appearance of symptoms is close and obvious. There is also the complication that commercial orange juices may look like orange juice and taste like orange juice, yet contain nothing but sugar, water, artificial flavoring, and food coloring. A reaction to ersatz OJ probably originates with one of the chemicals in the solution.

Berries are also notorious for their ability to trigger rashes—usually hives—in some individuals. Here, too, the link between cause and symptom is usually clear as is the appropriate response, which is not to eat whatever is causing the problem.

Meat

Meat, in and of itself, is not very likely to trigger hypersensitivity or allergic reactions. For one thing, it probably does not carry the parasites that, according to leading authorities, were pivotal in the evolution of the IgE immune response. However, the loss of parasites has been more than made up for by contemporary production practices in which animals and poultry are given various hormones and antibiotics. These substances remain as residues and carry risks for consumers. In addition, sanitary precautions in large-scale meat and especially poultry processing plants are haphazard, and government monitoring of the conditions under which meat is produced is extremely superficial. As a result it has been estimated that up to 50 percent of packaged chicken fryers sent out by some processors contain salmonella—bacteria capable of causing serious gastric symptoms.

Nor are the producers entirely to blame for marketing meat that can make you sick. Shellfish, for example, thrive under conditions where they are often likely to pick up and transmit microorganisms that can give you anything from a case of diarrhea to hepatitis A. And, once the product reaches the merchants' shelves, they may be disposed to treat it in various ways—the bright red color of beef in the meat display case is supposed to denote freshness, but often results from being treated with dye. Various kinds of preservatives are applied, more or less indiscriminately; some of them, such as sulfiting agents, are notorious for their ability to trigger irritant or allergic reactions, occasionally with fatal results.

In the case of processed meats—whether canned or preserved—additives or residues represent potential threats. Consult Table 11 to check on what the label tells you about additives and their potential for making trouble for you.

This has been one of the most difficult chapters for us to write, partly because diets are so diverse. Food is an essential part of cultures and lifestyles, which are highly variable. This diversity forces you, the sufferer, into a pivotal role. In our experience it is virtually always you, the patient, not your physician, who figures out what food or foods you are sensitive to. And, for the successful searcher, the most helpful tool is a carefully maintained food diary, a complete register of everything that you ingest—foods, liquids, medications.

Most doctors simply ask you to write down what you have eaten but, in our experience, that results in fragmentary and all-too-often illegible scrawls. To help you maintain your diary we offer Table 15 as a guide. Copy it and complete it carefully; if you do have a food sensitivity, it should be revealed in time unless your symptoms turn up so seldom that their cause is not likely to be revealed in any diary kept for only a limited period of time. Once you have identified the food—or additive or contaminant—responsible for your symptoms, consult the various "allergen-free" diets given in Appendixes G–K to help guide you away from it.

Points to Remember

In this chapter we discuss many of the reactions that food can elicit. True allergic reactions to food are much less common than hypersensitivity or irritant reactions: food itself is much less likely to cause problems than the coloring agents, stabilizers, and preservatives that have been added to it. Many of these

Table 15

Food Diary

Directions for Using the Food Diary

Fill out the Food Diary each evening preferably just before retiring. For the Symptoms section, if there were no symptoms, leave the spaces blank; if there were symptoms, indicate what they were (nausea, diarrhea, stomach pain, gas, hives, wheezing, etc.), when they appeared, how severe they were, whether they disappeared or persisted and got worse.

For the balance of the form, try to recall everything you ate or drank during the day and indicate by a check mark those you did ingest. Be particularly attentive to food additives (preservatives, dyes, flavor enhancers) since the bulk of gastric symptoms (allergic or irritant) originate from them.

At the end of the week record the number of checks for each item in the Total column at the right; then look for relationships between Symptoms and specific items consumed.

Summarize your analysis and your ideas about the causative agent or agents below:

Dates	Symptoms	Possible causes

(Duplicate Copies of This Table Before Using)

For_____Week of_____ to_____ , 19___
          (Name)

	Mon	Tue	Wed	Thu	Fri	Sat	Sun
Total							
*What were the symptoms?*___							
When did the symptoms appear?							
Morning___							
Afternoon___							
Evening___							
During the night___							
How severe were the symptoms?							
No symptoms shown___							
Mild___							
Moderate___							
Severe___							
What happened to the symptoms?							
Disappeared___							
Disappeared & returned							
Persisted___							
Persisted & got worse							

	Mon	Tue	Wed	Thu	Fri	Sat	Sun	Total
What did you eat?								
Grains or cereals (breads, pastries, breakfast foods, crackers, etc.)___								
Milk or milk products (ice cream, cheese, sour cream, cottage cheese, yogurt, etc.___								
*Eggs / egg products*___								
*Poultry*___								
Meats, fresh*___								
___								
___								
Meats, processed*___								
*Fish*___								
Shellfish*___								
___								
Vegetables Green, raw___								
Green, fresh, cooked___								
canned___								
Other, raw___								
Other, fresh, cooked___								
Other, canned___								
(Circle any of the above that were prepared by frying in oil; record brand name of oil, if known)___								
Fruits Citrus___								
Tomatoes___								
Berries___								
Melon___								
Other*___								

	Mon	Tue	Wed	Thu	Fri	Sat	Sun	Total
Snacks, including								
Candies								
Potato or other chips								
Dips								
Chocolate								
Nuts, nut butter, or nut oil for cooking								
Popcorn								
Chewing gum								
Other*								
Beverages, including								
Tea								
Coffee								
Cola/sodas								
Fruit drink								
Beer								
Wine (red or white)								
Other alcoholic drink								
What medications did you take, if any?								
Aspirin								
Cold or flu remedies								
Antibiotics								
Other*								
Did you (so far as you know) eat any of the following food additives?								
Preservatives								
Sulfiting agents								
Sodium benzoate and benzoic acid								
Sodium proprionate								
BHA or BHT								

	Mon	Tue	Wed	Thu	Fri	Sat	Sun	Total
Coloring								
Tartrazine (Yellow #5)								
Red								
Other*								
Enhancers and sweeteners								
Monosodium glutamate								
Saccharine								
Nutrasweet								
Spices*								

*Specify

materials are simply added to food to improve appearance, lengthen shelf life and thus boost profits. They have no food value.

Knowing how to read a package label is important. Be careful of package labels that claim they contain "pure" or "natural" contents. The terms are used indiscriminately and are essentially meaningless. It will pay you to be suspicious of everything you are about to consume. Carefully scrutinize the labels to see whether the food substance contains something that might be causing you trouble.

As an important element in ridding yourself of allergic or sensitive reactions to food or food additives, keep a diary. If you do this consistently and thoroughly, it will help to pinpoint the cause of your problem or make it easier for someone to help you.

CHAPTER 7

The Air You Breathe

Pollens, Dust, Dander, Mold, Pollutants

The air you breathe transports an impressive number of substances capable of provoking allergic or irritant reactions.

Allergic respiratory diseases—asthma and hay fever—trouble over 35 million Americans, or about 15 percent of the total population. Airborne substances trigger symptoms in the great majority of these individuals. In addition to those manifesting allergic reactions, countless other people display transitory irritant respiratory symptoms to airborne irritants.

Important Causes
of Respiratory Allergic Disease

The symptoms associated with hay fever are

1. Repeated sneezing, often 5–10 times consecutively, worse in the morning.
2. Eyes that water, smart, or itch.
3. Itching in the ear canals, throat, or roof of the mouth. (You feel that you have to run your tongue over or otherwise scratch the back of the mouth or soft palate.)

4. Dark circles ("allergic shiners") under the eyes.
5. Persistent watery nasal discharge.
6. Chronic nasal stuffiness, often associated with mouth breathing.
7. Scratching or repeated wrinkling or rubbing of the nose.
8. Unexplained nosebleeds.
9. Loss of taste of food.

Wheezing and shortness of breath accompanied by a dry or nonproductive cough are the usual symptoms of asthma.

The major airborne agents responsible for hay fever—allergic rhinitis—or asthma are:

Pollens
Molds
Animal danders
House dust

Pollens

Pollens, by all odds, account for the great majority of hay fever attacks. The good news about pollen-induced hay fever is that it is usually confined to a particular season of the year. Also on the good news side of the equation is the fact that recent advances in treatment have made effective management and control of hay fever possible without the substantial side effects that earlier medications carried. The bad news is that there are pollens capable of triggering hay fever floating around during much of the year, so that the relatively small number of individuals who are susceptible to more than one kind of pollen will be miserable during more than one season.

The season that hay fever hits corresponds roughly to the times that different types of plants give off pollen. Trees pollenate in late winter and spring, grasses in late spring and summer, weeds in late summer and fall. If you live in the midwestern part of the United States and if your hay fever hits in August and persists until the first frost, ragweed pollen most likely causes your sneezing and sniffling. If you reside in the mountains of Northern California and your symptoms show up in the spring, suspect Western Red Cedar pollen as the trigger.

Appendix B presents a map and table showing what plants cause hay fever, indicating when and where they are active in the continental United States and Canada. Consulting Appendix B will help you tie your symptoms to a possible cause or causes.

Your responses to the following set of questions will help you to decide if your symptoms are pollen-induced:

1. Are your symptoms seasonal?
2. Are they accompanied by an itchy palate or throat?
3. Are they worse in early morning or at night?
4. Are they worse out-of-doors?
5. Do they get better immediately after a rain?
6. Do they get worse on windy days?
7. Are they worse on days when the pollen count is high? (The weather page in most daily newspapers carries the pollen count.)
8. Do they get better when you are on vacation?
9. Are they worse when you mow the lawn?

If you answered No to three or more of the questions—especially those among the first four—chances are that your hay fever is not pollen-caused. Chapter 12 presents strategies for controlling pollens or other irritants originating outside the home. One tactic we do not recommend is the one Sally followed.

Sally suffered from allergies all of her life; the center of her universe was a box of Kleenex. Finally, in desperation, she moved to Arizona. What happened at the outset seemed miraculous; almost overnight her hay fever vanished. She was a little puzzled why the Phoenix phone directory had so many allergists listed in the yellow pages— but not for long. Two years later she herself was thumbing through those same yellow pages. Sally improved initially because she had managed to run away from the ragweed that had plagued her in Illinois. Within two years she had become sensitized to the Arizona pollens, especially sage, and her hay fever was back, full force.

Nor did Paul's attempted solution pay off.

Paul attacked his allergy to olive tree pollen aggressively by applying a chain saw to the olive tree in his yard. Yet, his symptoms persisted. He hadn't realized that olive tree pollen (and most others) can float for miles and there were many such trees nearby.

Seasonal, pollen-triggered hay fever can almost always be managed effectively with medication: mild, short-lived bouts usually respond to an over-the-counter antihistamine like Actifed; more severe or persistent symptoms yield to the intranasal steroids, Beconase and Nasalide. Antihistamines do cause drowsiness, so they should be used sparingly and those taking them should be especially careful about driving or working with potentially dangerous machinery.

Two prescription antihistamines, Seldane and Hismanal, are nonsedative and avoid these unpleasant side effects. Intranasal steroids (which do require a prescription) have no known serious side effects. To be maximally effective, treatment should be initiated a couple of weeks before your particular nemesis comes drifting in, and then the amount of medicine you use should be adjusted to the minimum needed to ward off symptoms. They can produce local irritation, may burn, and can cause nosebleeds. These complications, however, are minor and always reversible. Until quite recently, desensitization through the administration of allergy shots was the usual mode of treatment of moderate to severe hay fever. (After determining the exact cause of your symptoms through a series of scratch or prick tests, the doctor renders you less sensitive to it by injecting you with gradually increasing concentrations of the antigen responsible for your illness, thus building up your immunity to it. This procedure is costly, time-consuming, and carries some risks. We do not recommend it as a routine, first-line method of treatment.)

In instances in which exposure to pollens (or other airborne allergens) results in asthmatic symptoms, treatment strategies should be worked out in advance with your family doctor, possibly in consultation with an allergist. Asthma is evidently becoming more prevalent and asthma-linked deaths have been on the rise for the past decade and a half. It is a serious condition and one not to be trifled with.

Where your hay fever persists year-round, clearly the trigger holds a long-term lease on your environment. Molds, house dust, and animal dander are the prime causes of these chronic manifestations.

We spell out measures for controlling these antigens in Chapter 12. Beyond what we say there, note the following.

House Dust

House dust catches the blame, but dust mites— microscopic arthropods (members of the spider family) bearing names like *Dermatophagoides farinae* and *Dermatophagoides pteronyssinus*—are the principal antigens in it. Fortunately, mites can be kept out of your environment, but only if you control indoor temperature and humidity, follow a careful cleanliness regimen, and get rid of decor that harbors the pests.

Molds

Molds are microscopic fungi that live on dead plant or animal matter. They reproduce by releasing spores into the air and these spores, when inhaled, can produce respiratory allergic symptoms. Here again, environmental control is the key to successful avoidance of symptoms, and these procedures (and the places where mold grows) are also spelled out in Chapter 12.

It is not entirely clear what the actual antigen in mold spores is. This uncertainty has spawned an unfounded, eccentric, and damaging hypothesis about the relationship between mold and illness. Disciples of the so-called "Candida connection" (Candida—yeast—is one of literally thousands of varieties of mold) contend that people with some forms of allergies (as well as other diffuse, vague, and disabling symptoms) may harbor Candida or Monilia in their bodies. This colonization is said to bring about the release of certain products that, in their turn, trigger the complaints.

The Candida corps of practitioners claims that ordinary diagnostic methods fail to detect these infections and that treatment with antifungal antibiotics will put matters to right.

If you had the sort of internal yeast infection claimed, your family and friends would be in mourning. Yeast infections of the mouth, intestinal tract, or vagina occur often, but these areas are all considered external to the body. Treating some chronic condition said to be caused by an internal Candida infection with broad spectrum antibiotics is not only futile, but may well carry potentially serious and durable negative side effects.

Animal Danders

Animal danders make life miserable for many people. Actually dander (sloughed off scales of skin) represents only a part of the problem—animal saliva or urine that dries and becomes airborne contributes to respiratory distress when the particles are inhaled.

Antigens from cats and horses are especially potent, but other animals, including rats, dogs, birds, gerbils, hamsters, mice, and guinea pigs, do cause allergic reactions in susceptible persons. So do products

made from the animals—down comforters, wall hangings, rugs, fur apparel, and so on. You can best control allergic respiratory reactions to animals or their
products by getting them out of your environment and
avoiding those places where they are—or have been—
present. In practice this advice may be difficult to follow for several reasons. For example, travelers
smuggle pets into motel rooms. Second, newly acquired
houses or apartments often amount to warehouses for
the detritus left by pets of earlier occupants. Finally,
your hosts may not be completely forthcoming when
they assure you that Grover is an outdoor cat, neglect-
ing to add, "...except that when it rains we let the poor
thing in."

Not only can the pets themselves directly cause
you trouble; their foods, their medications, and their
mold-laden food and water dishes, or tanks, or cages
can also spell respiratory allergies. Dust from dry dog
food is known to have caused asthma, as has a powdered enzyme administered to combat canine pancreatic insufficiency.

Treatment strategies for chronic hay fever or for
asthma provoked by molds, dust, or animal dander
are essentially the same as those directed at the seasonal, pollen-caused form: Identify and studiously
avoid or eradicate the cause; counter minor episodes
with antihistamines; and treat more serious attacks
with intranasal steroids.

Since symptoms from these allergens can and do
occur year-round, desensitization through allergy
shots may sometimes be appropriate, although this
treatment should be weighed very seriously if asthma
is present.

Other Causes of Respiratory Allergic Disease or Hypersensitive Reactions

As we noted at the beginning of this chapter, the air you breathe picks up and delivers a myriad of particles capable of triggering temporary respiratory distress, either allergic or irritant in character. Table 16 lists a few of the substances you are likely to encounter that have the potential to cause you respiratory distress. In addition, see Chapter 13, which identifies allergy- or sensitivity-causing substances found in the workplace—and often in the home as well.

A Note About Air Pollution

The air in most American cities fails to meet federal health standards. Emissions from coal-burning power plants and internal combustion engines freight our air with ozone, carbon monoxide, nitrogen dioxide, sulfur dioxide, particulates, and lead. Although the long-term effects of these substances are not categorically known, there is considerable reason to believe that they may act individually or in concert to help sensitize, trigger, or intensify some chronic respiratory diseases, particularly asthma. They can also act as irritants, provoking transitory breathing difficulties as well as causing damage to the airways.

There are several points worth remembering about pollen counts and air quality measurements. The pollen counts and Pollution Standards Index (PSI) are given in parts per million—so many particles per million parts of air. These figures vary according to the time of day that samples are taken and the point where the sample is drawn. Thus, if you live in the

Table 16

Common Airborne Triggers of Respiratory
Allergic or Irritant Reactions

Products of combustion of
   Tobacco
   Wood
   Hydrocarbons (coal, gasoline, kerosene, diesel fuel,
      natural gas, propane, butane)

Fumes from
   Paints, varnishes, lacquer, shellac, mastics, adhesives,
      solvents

Plant products
   Orris root (a constituent of cosmetics)
   Pyrethrum (an insecticide constituent derived from a
      plant related to the ragweed family)
   Cottonseed and flaxseed (found in animal feeds,
      fertilizers, inexpensive upholstery, hair sprays, foods)

Household chemicals
   Dry detergents, soap powders, cleansers, waxes, air
      "fresheners", glass cleaners, bleaches, oven cleaners,
      insecticides

Aerosols
   Many of the hundreds of products delivered in pres-
      surized containers from paints to hair sprays to
      household cleansers have the capacity to trigger
      respiratory distress

Miscellaneous
   Perfumes, colognes, lotions, deodorants, body powders,
      other toiletries

---

inner city, where particulate concentrations tend to be high, and the sample reported in the newspaper is drawn away from the central city, where counts run lower, you may be at greater risk than the forecasters predict.

Second, the reports are usually presented categorically—the air quality is said to be healthful, marginal, or unhealthful and the pollen counts for grasses, trees, weeds, and molds are reported as low, moderate, or high. These judgments about the measurements are based on how "normal" people will be affected by the concentration of airborne allergens or irritants, but individuals with sensitivities may have much lower tolerance for irritants or allergens than ordinary folk. If you are smog-sensitive, your reaction to a "marginal" PSI reading may be equivalent to that of a non-sensitive person to an "unhealthful" PSI.

These statistics are usually offered as forecasts and they can err, just as weather predictions can and do. If wind conditions change, concentrations of pollens and pollutants will also change.

The point here is that the data you are being provided are based on extremely narrow samples, they are presented in such a way as to understate the risk potential to susceptible persons, and they can change substantially in a short period of time. Your best tactic is to correlate your symptoms with the reported conditions by keeping a written daily record, and then to develop defensive procedures based on your own experience. If you start experiencing symptoms when the PSI hits 60 (in the "healthful" range) then, when the forecast for tomorrow says "PSI 60," start doing what you need to do to stay healthy—keep indoors, don't do strenuous exercise, wear a mask, do whatever you need to do to avoid or prevent the onset of allergic or irritant-induced symptoms.

Points to Remember

The air you breathe is freighted with an array of naturally occurring and human-made particles that can spell trouble for the allergen or irritant-sensitive person.

The main "natural" allergens are pollens, mold, animal danders, and house dust; they can be largely avoided by applying the appropriate combination of environmental safeguarding measures, and the symptoms can be managed with medications. The principal human-made offenders are the result of the combustion of hydrocarbons and the increasing invasion of the environment by chemicals. Their effects, too, can be countered by avoiding exposure, instituting strict control measures, and where necessary, using protective devices. The chapters in Part 5 will tell you how to proceed in your various milieus.

CHAPTER 8

The Water You Drink

and Other Liquids

Water

Bottling and selling water that is advertised to be safe and palatable for drinking is something of a growth industry in the United States. Clear, sweet, pure drinking water from the tap is becoming a scarce commodity. According to a recent survey of supermarket shelves, a gallon of the bottled stuff can cost more than an equivalent quantity of gasoline.

Treated municipal water supplies are generally safe, but sometimes not fit to drink because they carry the disagreeable taste of chemicals that are used for purification or may otherwise invade the supply—herbicides, insecticides, or industrial waste products in particular. And since we continue to treat our lakes and streams as sewers, there is scant likelihood that the quality of what flows from the tap will improve in the foreseeable future.

In addition to H_2O itself, treated drinking water may, beyond whatever minerals and trace elements it contains, have added to it chlorine to kill harmful microorganisms, fluoride to prevent tooth decay, and other chemicals such as alum to clarify it. Despite the continuing controversy, none of the chemicals used in treatment is known to be harmful to humans, although chlorine does impart a distinctive and (to many) unpleasant taste. In fact, it may be this characteristic that has led to the phenomenal growth in sales of bottled water, home water filtration systems, and the gradual replacement of water by canned or bottled sodas as the thirst quenchers of choice.

In rare instances the public supply may carry toxic materials capable of causing severe, long-term health damage; arsenic concentrations in some California municipal water systems exceed recommended maximums and the Love Canal succeeded in compromising Niagara Falls' supply, but these are exceptions. Municipally treated water supplies are probably safe, even when unpalatable.

Untreated domestic water supplies arising from ground water—wells or springs—can carry a host of pollutants or contaminants capable of causing long-term disease, as well as much more quick-to-appear allergic or irritant reactions or infections.

For the most part, unsafe water may provoke gastric complaints in the short run—pain, nausea, diarrhea, cramps, fever, hepatitis. These symptoms arise principally from infections caused by bacteria or other microorganisms, such as giardia, that invade the water supply, are ingested, and do their mischief.

> There has been a moratorium on new building in one small Northern California town for the past decade. The reason? The underground water supply on which the residents depend has been contaminated by human waste released from privies, cesspools, and septic systems over the years. A sewage treatment plant was installed two years

ago, but the ground water still shows significant counts of coliform bacteria and its quality has not improved enough to meet minimal health standards. In the meantime the residents either boil their drinking water, buy it at the supermarket, or take their chances. Upset stomachs are commonplace in the town.

Other contaminants may make their way into the water supply from industrial wastes, particularly volatile organic compounds and the many exotic chemicals that are finding their way into factories and defense establishments. Housekeeping has not been one of the notable preoccupations of American industry, and many of these substances (identifiable by laboratory analysis) are quite capable of causing a wide array of complaints.

Even the plumbing, the pipes that carry the water, can cause health problems. Lead, copper, and (probably) plastic piping all make their little contributions to what we are drinking and, in the case of the metals, can and do produce profound long-term systemic health effects. Some historians go so far as to name lead—water pipes, dishes, and utensils—as one of the contributory causes to the fall of the Roman Empire. A few of our older houses still transport water through lead pipes; copper has been the material of choice for interior plumbing for the past several decades. Water carried through these pipes will bear traces of the metals. If you have copper pipes in your dwelling, never use the hot water faucet to deliver drinking water, and always let the cold water run a few moments before filling the glass, tea kettle, or ice cube tray.

Table 17
Contaminants Found in Domestic Water Supplies
and Their Potential Effects

Contaminant	Effect
Lead	Mental retardation
Arsenic	Cancer
Selenium	Birth defects
Pesticides, herbicides	Cancer, birth defects
Petrochemicals	Cancer
Bacteria	Infections, diarrhea

Water from underground sources can also contain radon, an odorless, tasteless gas that, when breathed for long periods of time and in sufficient concentration, is known to cause cancer. [Drinking radon-bearing water is not a health risk according the Environmental Protection Agency (EPA).] If your home has an undesirably high concentration of radon (*see* Chapter 11 and Appendix O for tests and strategies to follow) you may want regularly to test the water for radon. If your household water is found to be contributing significantly to the radon level in your home (this is not a particularly likely eventuality), you may want to consider installing a Granular Activated Carbon (GAC) filter to remove the radon. Such an installation costs upwards of $1000 initially, carries maintenance expenses, and poses some risks to the person doing the maintenance. Before undertaking any project involving removal of radon from your water supply you are encouraged to contact the EPA regional office nearest you. Their addresses and phone numbers are listed in Appendix G.

Industrial or agricultural discharges or waste are increasingly taking center stage as water supply contaminants. The list of substances is long and growing. Table 17 names some of the more common villains and indicates what their health effects are known to be.

Strategies for Getting Safe, Palatable Drinking Water

There are a number of options open to you to improve the safety and quality of your drinking water.

You can purchase bottled drinkinq water at the store or from local suppliers. This is an expensive solution and, unhappily, one that is not without its own risks. Some of the bottled mineral waters contain undesirably high concentrations of minerals, especially sodium, phosphorus, etc., which can cause health problems. They, like any other water supply, are also open to contamination, as the recent Perrier experience with recalling benzene-contaminated bottles demonstrates. And, one marketer of bottled "spring" water in a large California city was successfully prosecuted not long ago for misrepresentation when he was observed refilling the 5-gallon bottles from a garden hose attached to the city's (and his house's) water supply. (Interestingly, no customers complained that his stuff tasted like what they were paying handsomely not to imbibe.) If you choose this route, first be sure of your supplier. Second, read the labels. In Table 18, we include analyses of the composition of some of the nationally distributed brands of mineral water, and have identified as "not recommended" those with undesirably high concentrations of minerals. On the other hand, there are bottled waters that are low in salt, and some even contain desirable quantities of calcium. These are potentially beneficial and are highlighted in Table 18.

You can boil the water, which, if you do it long enough (20 minutes at least), will kill any microorganisms, but won't help the taste, is expensive, and adds up to being a nuisance.

You can use in-line filters. Here you have a variety of options; there are a multitude of firms that will supply and, where necessary, install water purifications systems for your domestic supply. These installations can be relatively simple—on the cold water line under the kitchen sink, for example—or extensive, treating the entire household supply. They can be set up to remove sediment, to deodorize, to precipitate minerals and soften the water, and to purify. Depending on your need, the costs can run from under $50 to well over $1000 for the initial installation. A do-it-yourself under-the-sink unit intended to deodorize and remove bad taste from an existing safe supply can be done for the lower figure; filters will have to be changed periodically and will represent an additional modest recurring cost. Suppliers are listed in the Yellow Pages under the Water Filtration and Purification Equipment heading.

You can use a gravity filter. This sort of arrangement involves having impurities and sediment removed as the water passes through a porcelain filter. This procedure is often used in developing countries where the water is known to be unsafe. However, the porcelain gravity filter is cumbersome, requires con-

Table 18
Content Analysis of Nationally
Distributed Mineral Waters

	Calcium[2]	Magnesium	Sodium[2]
Recommended waters			
1. Vittel Grande Source	202	36	3
2. Evian	78	23	5.5
3. Bartlett Springs	67	360	4.3
Not-recommended waters[3]			
1. Penafiel	574	198	333
2. Apollinaris	466	857	613
3. Golden Nectar	80	850	170
4. Vichy Springs	157	48	1095
5. A Santé	108	34	46
6. Mendocino	380	120	105
7. Crystal Geyser	12	3.1	130
8. Calistoga	80	3.4	128
Waters with minimal mineral content[4]			
1. Artesia			
2. Ozarka Spring Water			
3. Poland Springs Water			
4. Hawaiian Sparkling Water			
5. Alhambra			

[1]In general, waters that are recommended have desirable calcium and/or magnesium, but are low in sodium.
[2]PPM
[3]Waters that are "not-recommended" have in general more sodium than desired.
[4]These waters carry no recommendation, but we note the absence of beneficial minerals. They may, however, be safer to drink than tap water.

tinual monitoring, doesn't improve the taste, and is not particularly effective. The units are attractive, though, and make a nice conversation piece.

Outside the site of the ancient Roman baths in Bath, England stands a charming little fountain and statue that proclaims "Water Is Best." However, water is giving way to a host of other beverages (all water-based, of course) as thirst-quenchers of choice. The bulk of these substitutes carry some risk for allergic or hypersensitive individuals.

Sodas and Seltzers

These beverages—the colas, the uncolas, the rainbow of "pops"—are a mix of carbonated water (to give them their fizz), sugar or sugar substitutes, flavorings, dyes or coloring agents, and preservatives. Some of them also contain caffeine.

A standard, sugar-sweetened, 12-ounce container of soda gives you about 200 empty calories and, if you are susceptible to any of the freight of chemicals it carries, a chance to wheeze or break out in hives. The dyes, the sweeteners, and the preservatives are all capable of causing reactions; read the label of any soda or seltzer container carefully before drinking its contents. Keep in mind that it is still made up mainly of water, which is probably no purer or safer than the stuff you get from your own faucet. In addition, there is concern that drinking cola will increase your risk of osteoporosis because the phosphate-rich drink removes calcium from your body. The result? Thinning of bones over time, and easy fractures in old age.

Coffee and Teas

Coffee and tea can be "straight" or decaffeinated. Whether straight or neutered, they carry risks; caffeine is a stimulant and a bronchodilator (indeed, strong black coffee is sometimes given to relieve mild asthmatic wheezing). However, drunk to excess—more than 3 cups or 24 fluid ounces per day—it is associated with vascular, gastric, and cardiac problems in some persons. On the other hand, decaffeinated forms of coffee are reported to be associated with the development of certain cancers.

There has been a proliferation of "herbal" teas in recent years as people try to move away from caffeine consumption. Some of them combine a variety of herbs or other substances that can provoke symptoms in susceptible individuals.

> Bob and Iris wanted to cut down on their coffee drinking because they thought it was making them edgy. They bought several different types of herb teas to try out. Iris found that the varieties containing hibiscus affected her breathing and the peppermint varieties gave Bob heartburn.

Beer

Beer consumption in the United States has been on the rise for quite a while. It, too, provides you with a heavy dose of empty calories, some exposure to grain, hops, yeast, and sugar, and about three-quarters of an ounce of alcohol in the standard, non-"lite" form. All of the ingredients in beer are capable of provoking allergic or irritant symptomatology—perhaps especially the alcohol—which can also lead to gastric and organ damage.

Wines

By volume, wines contain about twice as much alcohol as beer. Saint Paul counseled "Take not water, but a little wine for the stomach's sake," but that was before domestic winemakers started adding sulfite to their vintages. Sulfite, a preservative, lengthens the shelf life of the wine materially. It is also a potent allergen, whose use on fresh vegetables has been banned, and causes mild to severe reactions in individuals having respiratory allergies, particularly asthmatics. It is also known to trigger gastric problems in some individuals. Most wine producers do treat their product with sulfite, and the label on the bottle will disclose its presence.

Spirits

Distilled liquors—gin, whiskey, vodka, brandy and the like—are anywhere from 40 to 50% alcohol. Some of them contain coloring materials, and most of them are distilled from grain so they carry the potential for causing allergic reactions. However, their main threat is found in the direct damage they do to the gastric and circulatory systems, and to the judgment and coordination of individuals, especially when the drinker knocks back two or three drinks after work and then gets behind the wheel of a car. Hard liquor is best left alone.

Fruit Juices

Fruit juices come either canned or frozen, undiluted or concentrated, or powdered. In addition to the fruit juice itself (and some fruit juices or powdered concentrates contain no fruit whatsoever, merely a cornucopia of chemicals), the container is likely to hold sugar or sweetener, preservatives, dyes, acid, and other chemicals. Here again, the best approach is to inspect the label carefully to establish the presence of ingredients that you know will cause you respiratory or gastric distress, and to remember that the product is mainly water—and if it is a concentrate, water from your own source at that.

Milk

We have discussed milk and milk-related allergic and intolerance problems more fully in Chapter 6. Americans consume a phenomenal quantity of milk and milk products, and the sad fact is that it doesn't do everybody good. As we have noted, a substantial number of people, especially those drawn from ethnic minorities—Blacks and Hispanics—and the elderly are hypersensitive to milk or milk products and experience gastric upset when they consume them. Apart from that, milk (which does contain important vitamins and minerals, including calcium) is also freighted with fat and cholesterol. If milk gives you digestive problems, avoid it; if you can tolerate it, drink the low- or nonfat variety. It will give you what you need from the milk without burdening you with the heavy load of calories and animal fats. Remember that there are many nonfat milk-derived foods that may be excellent sources of calcium and are low calorie—such as yogurt.

Points to Remember

So, where does that leave us? Not in a very good place, really. Most of the beverages we use as substitutes for water carry the potential for triggering hypersensitivities, many of them are nutritional disasters, and the alcoholic beverages also tend to cloud judgment and contribute handsomely to long-term health problems and the highway death and injury toll. Probably the best advice we can give you is to stick as close to water as possible; if the water in your home tastes or smells bad, treat it with the appropriate filtering system. If you have to use something else—social occasions are likely to force other choices—stick to beverages that you know are safe for you and come in containers that at least can be recycled and carry a refund. If you buy a mineral water, at least buy a good one!

CHAPTER 9

The Things You Touch or Are Touched By

Plants, Leather, Fur, Fabrics, Chemicals

Despite Madison Avenue's encouragement that we regard skin primarily as a showcase for adornment, or as a hallmark of sex appeal, our epidermis is in fact crucial to health and well-being. The skin is a vital organ, just like the liver, heart, or lungs. It carries out a number of key functions linked to survival—functions such as: sweating to help regulate body temperature and eliminate bodily wastes; protection from infection; and "holding us together."It also, through changes in coloration or rash, gives important clues about the internal state of the body.

Since the skin is such a large organ and the only one easily open to direct observation, defects, blemishes, and disfigurements are readily apparent. If you have a problem with your skin, you soon notice it or are quickly told of it by someone else.

Skin problems—rashes, eruptions, sores, scaling, cracking—can be caused by a large number of conditions. Diseases such as chicken pox, measles, scarlet fever, and rubella have characteristic rashes that serve as primary aids in diagnosis. Skin eruptions such as acne are sometimes associated with diet or hormonal changes. Some forms of malignancy, including basal cell cancer and melanoma, are likely to be first observed on the skin. Other skin problems—warts or infections, for example—are the results of viral or bacterial activity.

Although there are a wealth of possible reasons for skin disorders, direct physical contact with objects or substances that trigger a reaction is by far the main cause. Some of these reactions are classically allergic in character; others are the result of simple irritation.

Allergic Skin Disorders

Eczema and hives (urticaria) are the most common allergic skin conditions.

The cause of eczema is not definitely known; it is most often encountered in infants and young children. The skin outbreak is usually preceded and accompanied by a maddening itchiness. Some allergists believe that the compulsive scratching that accompanies the itching actually causes the eczema rash.

The character of the rash itself varies with the age of the victim. In infants it is likely to be "wet" and will appear on the back of the head, face, and in the creases in the groin and the arm and leg joints. In older children and a few unfortunate adults the lesion is less itchy, dry, and scaly and is ordinarily confined to the hands and lower arms, the lower legs, and behind the ears.

Eczema can be stubborn in some cases, but it is usually treated successfully by combining appropriate medication with a careful program aimed at avoiding contact with substances that seem to trigger or

Table 19
Treatment for Eczema

1. SEE A PHYSICIAN IMMEDIATELY if serious scratch marks, lesions, crusting, discoloration, or infection is present. (Infection often accompanies eczema and is effectively quelled by antibiotics.)
2. Control scratching, itching, and the spread of sores by trimming nails closely, avoiding tight, excessively warm, harsh fabrics, extreme temperatures, strenuous activities, harsh soaps, detergents, and petrochemicals. Apply Burow's solution, aluminum acetate, available over-the-counter at your pharmacy. Follow directions for use closely.
3. See your physician if symptoms persist. He or she will probably prescribe topical corticosteroids to control the lesions and antihistamines for the itching.
4. Bathe no more than twice weekly. Use tepid water, lanolin-free oils, gentle soaps; apply creams after bath to keep the skin moist; between baths use water-free cleansers like Cetaphil.
5. Identify and avoid any allergens or irritants (including food) that either trigger or intensify the rash.
6. AVOID allergy shots, which are ineffective for eczema and may provoke a reaction.

intensify the symptoms. Harsh soaps and lotions are especially to be avoided. Table 19 spells out what to do to manage eczema.

Hives are large, blotchy wheals—raised, inflamed areas of the skin. Hives, too, are itchy and they can turn up anywhere on the body.

Almost any substance is capable of causing hives in a susceptible person, but the most common triggers are foods (*see* Chapter 6), insect stings or bites, or coming in contact with any of a formidable list of

Table 20
Triggers for Hives

Type or category	Specific agents
Contact (cutaneous)	Too numerous to list
Diseases	Rheumatic disorders, hyperthyroidism, some malignancies
Drugs and medications	Penicillin, sulfonamides, aspirin; almost all other drugs possible
Food	Nuts, peanuts (legumes), eggs, berries, seafood (shellfish), tomatoes, milk, cheese, yeast
Inhalants (rarely)	Pollens, dust, mold, animal danders
Insects	Stings (honey bee, wasp, fire ant, hornet, yellow jacket), body material (cockroach, May flies), bites (Triatoma)
Food additives	Tartrazine, benzoates

substances. Table 20 names the more common substances capable of triggering hives.

To complicate matters a bit, note that hives are less often the result of an allergic reaction; in most instances, they reflect a direct response to an irritant. Whether or not the symptoms are allergic in character is largely immaterial because the management strategy in either case is the same; treat the symptoms and avoid the offender. Symptoms of hives and what to do about them are given in Table 21.

Table 21
Symptoms of Acute Onset Type of Hives

Primary

1. Intense itching (especially in areas with considerable nerve structure, such as the hands, feet, groin)
2. Wheals (raised, irregularly shaped red blotches) that show white in response to a fingernail or other object drawn over them

Secondary

If any of these secondary symptoms appear, seek emergency medical treatment AT ONCE).

 1. Difficulty with breathing
 2. Wheezing
 3. Hoarseness or thickened speech
 4. Constricted feeling in chest
 5. Nausea or vomiting
 6. Difficulty in swallowing
 7. Abdominal pain
 8. Weakness
 9. Confusion
 10. Incontinence
 11. Irregular or thready pulse
 12. Drop in blood pressure
 13. Bluish or purple coloration
 14. Loss of consciousness

For primary symptoms, take oral antihistamines (Seldane, Hismanal, Benadryl, Atarax); if symptoms persist for 48 hours, see your physician; avoid alcohol, aspirin, heat, exertion; do not take quinine, opiates, antibiotics, and certain vitamins like thiamine that can release allergic mediators directly.

Contact Dermatitis

Contact dermatitis can be expressed in a variety of ways and can be either allergic or non-allergic (irritant) in origin. It is a generic term applied to a broad group of skin irritations, rashes, or eruptions arising from contact with a substance responsible for producing symptoms by a susceptible person. Certainly the most notorious triggers of contact dermatitis are members of the Rhus group of plants, especially poison oak, poison ivy, and poison sumac. Upwards of 50% of Americans are sensitive to these plants.

Ed loves to work in his garden and considers his weekend mornings the best times of his life. He spends every hour he can spare spading, mulching, planting, weeding, pruning, harvesting, or just watching the progress of his beloved plants. However, since moving from Philadelphia to rural Kentucky, he has had to learn to garden with gloves and to be very, very careful. He had heard about the three-pronged leaf when he was a Boy Scout, but somehow came to believe that poison ivy was a disease only of children. He quickly learned otherwise. Within weeks of moving to Kentucky he developed the rash and the terrible itch that poison ivy imparts. Like most people, he made the mistake of scratching the rash, and that simply seemed to spread it. Ed couldn't figure out what was the matter, but it didn't take long for his wife to diagnose Ed's rash as poison ivy. By this time much of his body was affected and his face was so swollen he could barely see. His wife drove him to the emergency room where he was treated with steroids that rid him of the symptoms. By taking precautions, Ed is able to

Table 22

Triggers of Contact Dermatitis in or Around the Home

Trigger	Locale
Poison plants	
Oak, ivy,sumac	Out-of-doors
Plant products	
Balsam of Peru	Pharmaceuticals, foods, perfumed products
Cassia oil	Flavorings, perfumes
Citrus oil	Perfumes, medications, syrups, liquors
Colophony	Paints, varnishes, cosmetics, adhesives
Costus oil	Perfumes
Laurel oil	Pharmaceuticals, foods, perfumes
Oak moss oil	Perfumes
Metals	
Nickel	Jewelry (earrings, bracelets, watch bands, etc.)
Leather	Shoes, upholstery, apparel, watchbands
Rubber	Footwear, gloves
Cosmetics	Face powders, mascara, eye liner, cake make-up, powdered deodorants
Chemicals	Too many to list. Among the more common ones are formaldehyde, chromate, ethylenediamine, mercapto-benzothiazole, thiourams, paraphenyl-enediamine, plus ingredients found in many popular household products—soaps, waxes, polishes, cleansers, insecticides, paints, varnishes, etc.

continue with his cherished hobby, but he is careful about where he walks or puts his gloved hands.

Table 22 names the causes of contact dermatitis commonly found around the home. Occupational triggers are covered in Chapter 13.

Prevention and Treatment of Contact Dermatitis

Contact dermatitis can be a troublesome and stubborn condition. To care for it effectively you will need to:
- identify the cause
- treat the symptoms
- avoid further exposure to the irritant

Identifying the Cause of Your Contact Dermatitis

Chapter 4 offers a decision chart that will help you to identify the irritant responsible for your condition. In addition, you should answer the following questions:

Where is the rash located? This is often the best indicator of the likely cause. Thus, rashes on the eyelids or scalp are almost always caused by cosmetics, hairsprays, or shampoos; hand dermatitis can result from lotions, perfumes, worksite chemicals, or poison plants; when the earlobes, wrists, or fingers are involved, jewelry should fall under suspicion; and foot problems may result from one's own footwear (rubber or leather), or contact with symptom-producing plants.

Is the rash itchy? Painful? The presence of itchiness or pain will permit a narrowing down of possible triggers and also help reveal the nature of the underlying damage to the skin.

In what ways have you changed your routine of daily activities in the past 72 hours? Here take care to try to remember any variations from your ordinary daily routine, no matter how minor or innocent they may seem. Have you changed your job or job duties; taken on new or different responsibilities/tasks at home? had medical or dental treatment?; changed or started medications?; gone to a new hairdresser or barber?; etc, etc. Almost any change will expose you to materials you do not ordinarily touch, and virtually any material can precipitate a problem in a susceptible person.

Once you have identified a likely suspect or suspects, the next step in nailing down the cause is to have a patch test administered by an allergist or dermatologist. Most commonly, a dermatologist will apply a solution containing the substance believed to be responsible for the symptoms directly to the skin, covering the site with a patch. After a period of time elapses (usually 48 hours), the site is inspected and the skin's reaction, if any, is noted. A positive reaction will establish a diagnosis and point the way to treatment. (Patch tests are quite effective in identifying the causes of cutaneous problems, but are not infallible and the results should not be taken as gospel.)

Treating the Symptoms of Contact Dermatitis

The mode of treatment of the rash or lesions resulting from contact dermatitis depends on its nature, cause, and location. In the case of a mild, isolated reaction, if you know and avoid any further contact with the agent responsible, the rash will be self-limiting and will disappear within a few days. Whatever the nature of the rash, you should avoid scratching it because scratching will not only spread the rash but will make infection a distinct possibility. When itching is present, bathing in Aveeno or applying Calamine lotion will relieve it. Avoid Caladryl lotion. This contains Calamine lotion laced with Benadryl and may even make you worse.

> Steve had a widespread and unsightly inflammation of the skin. He was positive he was allergic to something. He saw several dermatologists, each of whom tried to convince Steve that his dermatitis might be psychogenic and self-induced from scratching. Steve didn't buy this even though they pointed out that virtually every part of his body was marred except for the unreachable mid-portion of his back. Steve did agree to a test, however, and had a cast applied to his left arm from fingertip to elbow. He was more than a little embarrassed when he returned to the doctor two weeks later. Although Steve had almost scratched his way through the cast, when it was removed, the skin underneath was clear.

In addition to controlling the itching and avoiding scratching you would be well-advised to avoid the use of topical antihistamines (lotions or salves) containing Benadryl because it can aggravate certain skin conditions. Also, avoid direct exposure to the sun, wear loose clothing, and entirely cut out or curtail the use of cosmetics.

Avoiding Further Exposure to the Irritant

Once it is identified, avoiding exposure to the irritant responsible for your symptoms should be easy, provided you remain alert and thoughtful.

LJ is a professor at a large university. A veterinarian, she is extremely fond of animals and has made a hobby of collecting earrings made in the shape of animals. When she reached her mid-forties she began developing severe swelling, redness, and pain in her earlobes. It was quickly established that she was allergic to the nickel found in inexpensive jewelry. She had to give up wearing any of her metal menagerie that contained nickel, but she hasn't abandoned her hobby; she still collects the animals, but only wears the sets made of more expensive materials that don't cause her discomfort.

Learn all of the places where the trigger affecting you is likely to be found. If at all possible, remove the offending substance (or, better, have someone else remove it) from your surroundings. If it cannot be entirely avoided, then take precautions to see that you do not come into direct contact with it. Use appropriate protective equipment—gloves, eye shields, coveralls, masks—without fail. If necessary, have your dermatologist, allergist, local health department, or the health and safety official at your place of employment, health maintenance organization, or OSHA help you to develop avoidance strategies.

Care of the Skin

The media are crammed with advertisements promoting all sorts of skin care products—lotions, emollients, cleansers, astringents, moisturizers, and so on. Skin care products rake in billions—high profit billions—for their manufacturers and distributors. Some of these products go so far as to be prominently labeled as "hypoallergenic." Don't believe it. There are no standards for defining the term. Manufacturers and packagers are left virtually free and seize the opportunity to label products as they choose. They choose terms that are likely to boost sales. Take Ivory soap ads. Ivory, says Procter and Gamble, is safe for baby's tender skin, implying that it is soft, gentle, soothing. No way. Ivory soap contains lye, and in both lab tests and clinical experience has been found to be about the harshest and most irritating soap you can use. Use Ivory on your infant with eczema and watch the eczematous lesions blossom. (As a matter of fact, one of the authors has found Ivory suds to be an extremely effective herbicide.)

You can be kind to your skin without having to spend a fortune at the pharmacy. Here are the basics of good skin care.

- Use cosmetics sparingly, if at all. If you use them, they should be applied with cotton or a Q-tip, not your fingers, and special care should be taken to keep them out of your eyes.
- Be careful about using hair dyes. If you know you are sensitive to some of them, check with a dermatologist before using.
- Use mild soaps like Dove.
- Use a sunblocker or sunscreen, but only if you are not sensitive to the special chemical ingredients it contains. (Recent research indicates that a low number blocker—10 or 15—is as effective as the higher numbered and proportionately more expensive ones.)
- Wear plastic gloves when doing the dishes, or when using cleansers, solvents, and the like.
- Wear clothes that do not irritate the skin. Loose-

fitting, untreated cotton is safest; wools, poly-
esters, and fabrics treated to be wrinkle-resistant
or flame-retardant are the worst.

Points to Remember

Most people at some point or another in their lives
will experience a dermatitis triggered by something
that they have touched, or have somehow been brought
into contact with.

The good news is that most such episodes are
minor, isolated, and self-limiting. They can be treated
successfully in the great majority of instances, leave
no scars, and can be kept from recurring by identifying and studiously avoiding the agent or agents
responsible for the rash.

The bad news is that such a dermatitis may keep
you from trying to help the skin out by using beauty
preparations or adornments. But having beautiful,
clear skin, though certainly desirable, represents a
culturally defined ideal, and one that tries to ignore
the fact that, over a lifetime, the skin changes.
Wrinkles, spots, and folds inevitably show up; accepting them serenely as part of life's cycle will keep you
from emulating Ponce de Leon's painful and fruitless
quest.

PART 5

CREATING AND MAINTAINING ALLERGEN AND IRRITANT-FREE ENVIRONMENTS

CHAPTER 10

Establishing
and Maintaining
a Sound, Safe Diet

*Including Discussions of Vitamins, Fads,
Avoiding Word Traps Like "Natural,"
"Organic," "Artificial," and so on...*

The food you eat—your diet—can threaten your
health in two ways. As we noted in Chapter 6, some
foods or food additives may provoke allergic or irritant reactions in you. Depending on the trigger and
person involved, these reactions can range from mild,
short-lived annoyances to chronic and life-threatening assaults. In addition to, and more far-reaching in
its adverse health effects than its ability to cause allergic or allergic-like symptoms, food ranks as
America's most abused substance. As a nation we gob-
ble up too much of the wrong kind of food. The result
—an epidemic incidence of overweight and obesity,
clogged arteries, diet-linked cancers, and a host of
other food-associated complaints.

Rich played minor league baseball just long
enough to realize that he couldn't hit a curve ball.
In the minors he got in the habit of eating huge

139

breakfasts—orange juice, half a dozen eggs over easy, bacon or sausage, hash browns, toast with lots of butter and jam, milk, coffee laced with cream and sugar. Rich is 29 years old. His cholesterol level hovers around 325 and this statistic has led to some bitter arguments between him and his wife, Renee, a public health nurse, who knows the risks of high cholesterol and constantly tries to get Rich to eat more sensibly and moderately. Rich complains that Renee is trying to starve him, that he needs to feel full when he gets up from the table, and what she serves him saps his strength and energy.

Dealing with Allergic or Irritant Reactions to Foods

To be safe from allergic or irritant reactions to foods, food additives, or food contaminants, you must:

- Identify the trigger or triggers
- Avoid the triggers scrupulously
- If you react severely, carry appropriate medication with you at all times.

Part 3 spells out the tactics you can use to identify the foods, food additives, or contaminants responsible for your symptoms. Chapter 6 names the major triggers. An elimination diet and various "allergen-free" diets appear in the Appendices.

Charlene reacts violently to alcohol in the most minute quantities and in any form. She has to be extremely careful about what she eats or drinks. Mostly she prepares her own meals but, whenever she eats out she grills the food preparer intensely about everything that went into the dishes. She learned this lesson a few years ago when she ate a piece of cake that contained vanilla extract. This particular extract was 40 percent alcohol and before Charlene had eaten half of her piece of cake she was choking and gasping for breath. The timely use of an ANA-kit saved her a trip to the emergency room that time.

If you react severely to food or food additives—breathing problems, swelling of mucus tissue in the mouth, giddiness, widespread hives—you should develop a procedure to follow if you are inadvertently exposed to whatever it is that causes your symptoms. This procedure should be worked out in consultation with your allergist or family physician. In addition, if the symptoms are potentially life-threatening, you should:

- Wear Medic-Alert identification (*see* Appendix N for information on registering with Medic-Alert).
- Carry appropriate medication at all times. (Check regularly to be sure the medication is not too old to be effective. Devote some time on your birthday to carry out this review.)
- Train family members or others who are likely to be called on to help as to what they should do in an emergency. They should be able to recognize the symptoms, know what first aid measures to apply, how to administer any medications or drugs, and how to summon emergency medical care. One good way to acquire these skills is to complete an American Red Cross First Aid course that covers rescue breathing, CPR, and first aid for injuries and shock.

Table 23
Complications and Risks Associated with Obesity[1]

1. High blood pressure
2. Increased incidence of strokes
3. Reduced tolerance for exercise
4. Chronic obstructive pulmonary disease—emphysema
5. Inability to stay awake (narcolepsy)
6. Skin infections (boils)
7. Arthritis
8. Premature death

[1]Obesity is defined as weighing more than 10% over your ideal body weight. Your physician or HMO will have tables that provide the figures.

The Long-Term Implications of Food Abuse

Food or food additives can provoke a variety of allergic or hypersensitive reactions. The reactions appear quickly and, in most instances, soon fade away with no lasting ill effects. Food abuse can have an entirely different, but no less dangerous, set of consequences. These consequences can be persistent and pernicious. Being overweight or obese is a major health risk. Some of the complications of being overweight are listed in Table 23. "You can never be too rich or too thin" may overstate the case a bit—at least when it comes to thinness—but recent evidence indicates that even being a small amount overweight carries significant negative long-term health implications. Moreover, being overweight, in our experience, seems to exacerbate symptoms associated with allergic disease, especially asthma and vascular complications.

Being overweight is almost invariably the result of consuming more food than the body needs. The extra groceries wind up as fat deposits that our marvelously complex and efficient bodies produce. Give the body too much and it will find a place to store the excess—invariably at sites where it is as obvious as it is unwelcome.

Diets, dieting, and weight loss schemes are a major industry in the United States. Not a few of them are laughably implausible; some are potentially dangerous; some guarantee miracles; a few of them are well-conceived; most of them cost serious money; and none of them succeeds completely. This should come as no surprise when the dieter has to confront so much advertising devoted to promoting the sale and consumption of foods—advertising that is reflexively extravagant and one-sided in its representations.

We do not have yet another weight loss scheme to offer. We can line out what represents a well-rounded diet, one that contains the elements you need and cuts out much of what is bad for you. We can't regulate what or how much you consume; you, yourself have to do that and learning new habits and limits is terribly difficult.

A Sound Diet

How much you ought to eat depends on a number of factors—age, sex, and level of activity. Food value is most often expressed in terms of calories. A calorie is the quantity of energy required to raise the temperature of one kilogram of water one degree Centigrade. The caloric value of a given quantity of food—

usually expressed as a serving—is represented as 'Cal' on its container. Many up-to-date cookbooks also provide tables of this information. For older people or people in sedentary occupations, 2000 calories per day of the right kinds of foods is enough; children, and people in physically demanding occupations, may require a higher daily input.

What you ought to eat—or not eat—is a more complicated story. We all need sufficient quantities of protein, fat, carbohydrates, and fiber, plus vitamins, trace elements, and minerals in our diet. The required quantities may come from a variety of sources. In the United States, there is a well-practiced tendency to overload on meat proteins, fat, and carbohydrates, and to slight fiber, foods containing vitamins, and minerals. Our thoughts on what constitutes appropriate elements for the principal meals follow.

Breakfast

Breakfast, despite what you have been told, may not be the most important meal of the day. In fact, a light breakfast is to be preferred to stuffing yourself full of the traditional eggs, bacon, and pancakes, or to the wolfing of quick-fix products that are mainly chemical concoctions. The essential components of breakfast should be fruit and grain. You can get them any way you want, but you should avoid products heavily laced with sugar and be wary of those labeled as "natural" or instant. Instant breakfast bars, for instance, provide a lot of calories, but they also carry too much salt, preservatives, and far, far too much fat. If milk is part of the breakfast menu, make it the low-fat variety—skim milk. That way you'll get the calcium you need. If you have to have caffeine, tea or coffee in moderation are OK, but skip the cream and sugar.

In many households, part of the morning ritual is to stoke up on pills. We believe that pills—vitamins, "quick energy" or food supplements—are more than likely a waste of time and money, and they can be dangerous.

Joanne thought that body-building vitamins would help her cross-country skiing. She paid handsomely for that attempt at self-improvement. She didn't read the label, and so failed to realize that the pills she bought were only a chemical preparation of degraded milk products—and Joanne is exquisitely sensitive to lactose.

As we often say, knowing what you are taking into your body is half the battle. Turn yourself into a label-reading junkie. Chapter 6 tells you how to read labels effectively, and also points out what labels frequently don't tell you, which is often considerable. Efforts to reform package labeling are under way, but are being hampered by incomplete knowledge of just which and how much of each of the various vitamins, minerals, etc. is required to maintain health, and also by opposition from the food industry, which believes that its responsibility is to its stockholders, not its customers.

Lunch

In many cultures the noonday meal is the big one and is followed by a brief nap. This is a sensible way to live, but unlikely to become popular in this country where school or work are interrupted by a cruelly short lunch break. That constraint encourages people to eat in fast-food establishments, and fast-food establishments are inclined to dish up meat on a bun, french fries, and a shake or their equivalents. This is a banquet swimming in fat and bristling with calories. That quintessential lunch carries 1200 calories, 50 grams of fat, too much sugar, and virtually no fiber. Fastfood merchandisers agreed to provide dietary information to their patrons some time ago, but only one of the scores of chains has so far lived up to the promise.

For lunch, you will be well-advised (unless you are a growing child or pregnant) to avoid meat altogether. Concentrate instead on fruit, vegetables, and grain. A salad bar, easy on the dressing, makes better sense. If you must have meat, think lean. This is fairly hard to do in a "burger place" where the fat content of the meat may run as high as 35 percent.

Snacking

One important reason for the American problem with obesity is snacking. We provide breaks or recesses, morning and afternoon, to offer relief from the routine of work or school. Many use these breaks to grab a snack—candy bars, cookies, cake, a soda. A classic cola and a bag of potato chips can load you up with 500 calories, a lot of fat and salt, and no food value worth mentioning—the proverbial empty calories. If you must snack (and you ought to think twice about whether or not you need to), an apple or other piece of fruit, some raisins, or trail mix (if it is safe for you) are much to be preferred from the nutritional standpoint. The most vigorous snacking takes place in the evening, either before dinner over drinks, or after dinner during TV commercial breaks. If you can resist snacking and drastically limit your consumption of alcoholic beverages or sugar-loaded sodas, you will be doing yourself a major favor.

Meg is 32 and pretty—and plump. Actually she is five feet one inch tall and weighs in at 220 pounds. Each morning on the way to work and each evening on the way home from work, she stops at the corner Seven-Eleven and buys a giant soda to go. She sips while she does her work or while she fixes her vegetarian dinner. Meg is very conscious of the dangers from the fat and hormones and antibiotics that lurk in meat. She chooses not to recognize that those giant potions of sugar and chemicals in her soda cup give her about 800 empty calories every working day.

Alcohol is, of course, the ultimate dietary menace, loading you with calories while wreaking organic damage that can be considerable over time. A couple of 12 ounce bottles of beer on the way home from work —or shots or glasses of wine—carry about 600 calories. Period. Unless you want to count the sulfite.

Dinner

If we were sensible, dinner would be taken at midday, but in the US, it is usually eaten early enough in the evening to encourage postprandial snacking. Holding off the dinner hour until eight in the evening or thereabouts will help curb this tendency. Dinner should include grain, vegetables (cooked and/or raw), and protein (meat, fish, or other source). Limit oils and fats (in sauces, salad dressings, meat, chicken skin). If you must have something alcoholic to drink with dinner, wine is preferable to beer or a mixed drink. Note that some TV dinners, those bastard handmaidens of high tech cookery, are brimming with fats. We remain mystified at the apparent willingness of people voluntarily to prepare what amounts to airline meals—and then to eat them.

The "Natural" Myth

When it comes to food, we have permitted Madison Avenue to persuade us that "natural is synonymous with "good." Consider. Salt is natural, but it wreaks havoc with blood pressure; fat is natural, but too much of it is associated with heart attacks and strokes. Examine the package label of almost any product billed as natural and, when you get to the fine print, you're likely to find all sorts of chemical surprises—dyes, stabilizers, preservatives, flavor "enhancers." Natural is simply a word that has come to suggest that the product it is attached to exists in some pure, unadulterated state. In that sense almost no food that you can buy is natural; adding the word to the package somehow saddles us with the belief that these products are better for us. There are no limits on just how the word may be used and, correspondingly, there are no limits on how food manufacturers and distributors are willing to use it.

> Karen feeds her two year-old daughter 'natural' raw cow's milk because she does not want the child exposed to hormones and antibiotics that show up in regular milk. (The dairy vending the raw milk certifies that it does not treat its herd with hormones or antibiotics.) The child is made seriously ill by the salmonella bacteria that turn up in one batch.

Table 24
Constituents of an Ideal Daily Diet[1]

Elements[2]	Infants	Children	Adult Males	Adult Females
Protein (g)	13.5	16–28	45–63	46–50
Vitamin A (µg)	375	400–700	1000	800
Vitamin D (µg)	7.5–10	10	10	10
Vitamin E (mg)	3	6	10	8
Vitamin K (µg)	5–10	15–30	45–80	45–65
Vitamin C (mg)	35	45	60	60
Thiamin (mg)	.3	1.0	1.8	1.1
Riboflavin (mg)	.5	.9	1.5	1.1
Niacin (mg)	6	12	20	15
Vitamin B6 (mg)	.4	1.1	2.0	1.5
Folate (µg)	25–35	50–100	150–200	150–180
Vitamin B12 (µg)	.5	1.4	2.0	2.0
Calcium (mg)	400-600	800	1200	1200
Phosphorus (mg)	400	800	1200	1200
Magnesium (mg)	40-60	80-170	270–350	280
Zinc (mg)	1–2	2–10	10–12	10–12
Iron (mg)	6–10	10	10–12	15
Copper (mg)	0.2	0.4	1–2	1–2
Iodine (µg)	40–50	70–120	150	150
Selenium (µg)	10–15	20	40–70	45–65
Fiber (g)	—	—	12–15	12–15

[1]These are average values and represent only a rough guide.
[2]g = grams, mg = milligrams, µg = micrograms.

Arriving at a Safe, Sound Diet

Learning to eat sensibly and moderately is no easy task. Most people know what they ought to eat—but eating right requires time, effort, and the willingness to suspend the wrong-headed attitudes and prejudices that people attach to eating. To formulate a sensible diet for yourself, we suggest you start by keeping an exact and complete record of what you eat—keep a diary for a week. At the end of each day, record everything you have eaten or drunk that day and note the number of calories, the grams of salt, protein, calcium, fiber, and percent of average daily requirements of vitamins, trace elements, and minerals that the day's input amounted to. At the end of the week, aggregate what you have done and use the information to make adjustments to what and how much you consume. Table 24 recommends an ideal daily diet and provides you with data that will let you calculate how your daily intake compares with the recommended figures.

Points to Remember

Foods and food additives can provoke distressing reactions in some individuals but, on balance, the more serious problems come from eating too much of the wrong kinds of food. Even modest levels of overweight are associated with a variety of respiratory, vascular, coronary, and organ diseases, as are diets high in animal fats and cholesterol.

We have set forth a no-fads, sound, sensible diet plan in this chapter, and we hope that you will give it a try; we hope, too, that if food is associated with allergic or irritant reactions where you are concerned, you will take the trouble to seek out the offender and then bend serious effort to avoiding it—the best and virtually only recourse you have to food-linked allergic or hypersensitive conditions.

CHAPTER 11

Building a Safe House

This chapter is intended for all those who plan to build or remodel their own homes. Unfortunately, relatively few Americans live in accommodations where they have had the opportunity to exercise control over the materials that went into them because most people in the United States either occupy dwellings that were previously owned or rent them from a landlord. Even the bulk of new housing is built on speculation, carried out by developers who acquire a tract of land and erect residences on it in the hope that they will be able to sell the units at a profit.

What goes into the making of a house depends on the area of the country in which it is to be built—styles and construction strategies vary from one part of the country to another. In colder climates, for instance, the tendency is to start with a basement and to keep the structure itself relatively compact with an essentially vertical orientation. In the Sunbelt states, where heating and heat loss are not such important considerations, typical floor plans are inclined to be more horizontal or spread out. Each type of dwelling can present problems to individuals with allergies or hypersensitivities.

151

Geography also has much to do with the materials that actually go into a structure. The availability of materials and local customs and taste may well dictate the materials used for the exterior. Wood, stucco, brick, earth, stone, concrete, or metal may be seen to predominate from one locality to another. And for the most part, these traditional materials in their unadulterated form are not apt to trigger allergic or irritant reactions. The trouble is much more likely to originate with exposure to new, manufactured products or to chemicals used in the final or finish stage of construction.

If you are planning on building a new home, or adding on to or remodeling an existing home, your approach to the construction will be determined by your status with regard to allergies or hypersensitivities. If you react to substances contained in building materials and you know what they are, simply do not allow them to be used in the new construction. (There are substitutes available for almost any material at all that might trigger problems.) If you or any member of your family has a history of allergy or hypersensitivity that is expressed in respiratory or cutaneous symptoms (hay fever, asthma, eczema, contact dermatitis, hives), then it may be prudent to observe some precautions, both during the building process and in the choice of materials to be used.

In planning your new or remodeled dwelling, it may be quite sensible to consult with your allergist about what specific materials to avoid and then seek out an architect, contractor, and builder who makes a specialty of designing and erecting houses that are as free as possible from such harmful materials. Since this specialty is new and rare, you may be obliged to do considerable canvassing to find people with the desired knowledge and skills.

When you do locate the right people, brace yourself for two additional problems. First, finding suitable substitute materials will, in some instances, be difficult and time-consuming, and your costs will run 25–50% higher than those you would incur if you used conventional materials and techniques. Even so, your eventual savings in medical costs and in reduced physical and psychological stress ought, over time, to buy back much of the added initial cost and inconvenience.

Second, the incidence of sensitivity to construction materials is not definitely known. Although the media carry almost daily accounts of individuals reported to react to any of the hundreds of substances employed in the building process, the overall percentage of the population having such susceptibility is probably quite low.

Thus, although we cannot catalog all of the materials that go into the making of a house, we have identified, and listed in Table 25, the most important such materials, products, or substances employed at various stages of the construction process—materials that are known to cause allergic or hypersensitivity problems. The list makes no claim to being complete; a number of materials that provoke mild problems in a few individuals have not been cited, and, of course, there is a constantly expanding array of manufactured building products and chemicals, some of which will no doubt be found harmful down the road.

Along with the symptom-producing materials, we have identified the more common symptoms they trig-

Table 25
Irritants or Allergens Found in Building Materials

Irritant or allergen	Symptoms caused	Uses	Where found	Alternatives
Wood dust and wood resin vapors (Western red cedar, California redwood, other conifers)	Hay fever, asthma	Paneling, siding, decking, studs, sheathing	Interior or exterior walls, walls, decking, roof	Use well-seasoned wood; seal with non-irritant finish
Cement, mortar, and taping "mud"	Respiratory problems from dust; contact dermatitis from chromate	Foundation walks and driveways, drywall	Foundation, interior walls, other concrete or sheetrock uses	No substitute for concrete; use woods, tiles, plaster in lieu of drywall
Wood treatments, especially pentachlorophenyl, insecticides, fungicides	Respiratory and skin irritations	Wood preservative	Treated lumber (peeler cores, mud sills, studs, sheathing, roof shakes)	Use untreated lumber or apply safe preservatives like natural finishes or coatings
		Binding agent in drywall	Interior walls	Solid lumber, lime plaster, "natural" sheetrock
		Binding agent in timber products; plywood, chipboard, particle board, imitation wood paneling	Subfloor, interior and exterior walls, roof sheathing, cabinets, furniture, shelving,	Use solid lumber or where appropriate hardwoods, metal, glass
Formaldehyde (Vapors, resins, and fumes)	Respiratory or skin irritation; headache; nausea; fatigue	Fabrics (drapes, carpets, upholstery, wrinkle or stain resistant, flame retardant fabric	Synthetic carpets, drapes, upholstery, wall coverings, bed covers and bedding	Hardwood or tile flooring; cotton or other natural and untreated fibers; cork
		Adhesives, glues, and mastics hanging wallpaper, assembling furniture, caulking, and weather sealing	Installing wall and floor tiles	Employ older style materials dedicated to these uses

154

(continued...)

Table 25 (*continued*)

Irritant or allergen	Symptoms caused	Uses	Where found	Alternatives
Synthetic finishes (petrochemical or urethane varnishes, paints, stains, sealants, thinners, strippers)	Respiratory; cutaneous; headache; nausea	Covering or stripping exposed surfaces	Floor, walls, ceiling, furniture	Avoid petrochemical products containing urethane, epoxy resins, chloride; use water-based finishes, linseed or other oils, beeswax polish; use hard woods, cork, matting, or untreated natural fibers to cover walls
		Floor and wall tiles	Floor, walls	Use hardwoods, cork, tile, naturally occurring untreated fibers
		Electrical fixtures	Walls	Use ceramics
Polyvinyl chloride (PVC)	Respiratory, cutaneous	Plumbing pipes and cements	Subfloor and walls	Hard to avoid and minimally dangerous once in place; use copper for hot water
		Wallpaper	Walls	Use paper wall covering; install with wheat or other nonsynthetic paste
		Imitation wood paneling	Walls, ceiling	Avoid use; substitute hardwood, tile, cork, naturally occurring untreated fibers
Plastics, polyurethane	Respiratory, cutaneous	Foam filling in mattresses, pillows, furniture, upholstery, carpet pad	Furniture, bed, under carpeting	Polyurethane, in addition to offgasing, is a serious fire hazard; substitute cotton, kapok, or use furniture that is not heavily upholstered—hardwood, string, cane, etc.
Acrylics (Acrylic acid)	Respiratory, cutaneous	Substitute for glass	Windows, table tops, floor pads for furniture	Use glass where possible

ger, where they are encountered, and materials that can be used in their stead.

Foundation

Foundations are usually built of concrete that has been strengthened with structural steel ("rebar") and, where posts and piers are employed in lieu of a perimeter foundation, wood.

Rebar is not known to cause problems. If you are a do-it-yourselfer, cement dust can trigger respiratory problems, wheezing, and skin irritation. Avoid these problems either by having the concrete delivered ready-mixed (much easier and less labor-intensive, but more expensive) or by wearing a dust mask, gloves, and long sleeves and trousers when mixing the concrete. (Note that the cement is the problem; the finished product, concrete, is not known to cause reactions in and of itself.)

Wood foundation material may cause problems. Some people react to sawdust itself (if you do, wear a mask) or to resins in the wood, notably those produced by the several varieties of cedar, redwood, and other conifers. When the resin is the trigger, usually well-seasoned or recycled stock in which the resin has had time to dry out will ordinarily be safe, although cedar resins are persistent and you may have to substitute another type of lumber for it.

In addition, much foundation material is chemically treated to preserve it, making it less vulnerable to moisture and to insects, the two principal enemies of wood. Chemically treated posts placed on concrete footings and piers that support the structure are usually impregnated with pentachlorophenol, long-lasting insecticides like lindane and dieldrin, and with fungicides. These supports (the round posts are called "peeler cores") have a characteristic greenish-gray coloration. The chemicals trigger severe rashes, respiratory difficulties, or gastric symptoms in some individuals. Avoid using them if possible (*see* Table 25 for substitutes and safer methods of treatment). Note, too, that most mudsill stock is white fir that has been pressure-treated with pentachlorophenol.

At one time creosote was widely used for the preservation of wood. Its use has now been outlawed (it is carcinogenic and produces severe and widespread skin reactions in susceptible individuals), but it still turns up and should not be used in construction. Used railroad ties, which are popular material for the making of garden headers, outdoor planters, or terrace walls, are especially likely to be saturated with creosote or other dangerous preservatives. We do not recommend the use of such railroad ties in your home vegetable garden.

Floor

In some parts of the country, the floor may be nothing more than a steel-reinforced concrete slab. For the most part, though, the floor consists of joists, heavy timbers with, usually, a plywood or other form of manufactured lumber laid atop them. Then, after the joists are positioned and the subfloor laid, insulation will be placed between the joists, with the insulation itself often then covered with yet another bottom layer of thinner, manufactured wood.

Joists are usually untreated fir or pine; as already noted, these conifers carry resin that can be an irritant, so use only well-seasoned stock (somewhat more difficult to work with than the ordinary green timber supplied by lumber yards) or substitute hardwoods. (Some authorities argue that green lumber is better to work with because it produces less dust.)

Subflooring is usually made of manufactured wood —plywood, particle board, or chip board. Plywood consists of thin sheets of wood that has been bonded (glued) together under pressure in an opposing grain or laminated pattern to give it strength. It is sold in standard 4 x 8-ft. sheets in various thicknesses and grades, and its use has greatly speeded (and homogenized) home construction.

All manufactured woods are bonded with resins containing formaldehyde, a substance that causes skin irritation, respiratory problems, headache, nausea, and giddiness in an appreciable number of individuals. Plywood is bonded with phenolformaldehyde, which is somewhat less noxious than the other formaldehyde resins.

Particle board, chip board, flake board, and other manufactured "woods" formed out of fibers are somewhat more recent developments in the construction industry. They utilize what were once essentially waste products; by treating these waste bits of material with resins under heat and pressure, a product is created that competes with conventional plywood—it is in fact much cheaper, though far less durable and far harder to work with.

Particle, chip, and flake board contain a number of potentially harmful chemicals, urea formaldehyde resin being the most common and dangerous ingredient. These products are risky to handle, and release formaldehyde vapor, which can persist for long periods of time. Their use is not recommended.

Some manufacturers produce "low emission" formaldehyde products—primarily plywood—and these may be acceptable substitutes.

Walls and Ceiling

Exterior walls can be made of earth, stone, brick, wood, metal, concrete, or stucco. Brick, earth, and stone are relatively benign; sawdust and resin fumes from some woods, as we have seen, can trigger respiratory problems. Metal siding with, usually, baked-on enamel finish is ordinarily not troublesome, but dust from the cement or mortar used in concrete, brick work, and stucco can cause skin irritation or respiratory problems.

The exterior wall will ordinarily have a moisture barrier underlying it—black felt paper or more recent products like Tyvek or Typar. They are not known to cause allergic or hypersensitivity reactions.

Interior walls and ceilings, these days, are usually formed of dry wall (sheet rock or plasterboard which is phosphogypsum sandwiched into large paper-covered sheets 4 x 8 or 4 x 10 ft. in various thicknesses) cut to size and nailed to studs (vertical 2 x 4s) or rafters. Insulation in the form of rolls, pads, or pellets fills in the space between interior and exterior walls.

Both the unfinished interior wall and the insulation carried between exterior and interior wall can represent a source of trouble. Formaldehyde is used to bond the paper to the plaster core of dry wall and to cement the gypsum particles together so the interior wall can emit vapors from the adhesives with respiratory problems and eye and nose irritation being a common result. The gypsum dust that results from cutting sheet rock, hanging it, taping it, and texturing it also represents a potent respiratory irritant. When working with dry wall, use a mask. In addition, since the chromate in the "mud" used in taping and texturing drywall is a potent trigger of contact dermatitis, wear gloves when working with it and, if necessary, give your hands a protective coat of petroleum jelly.

> Phil was remodeling his home and working extensively with a mud used in texturing the dry wall. He did not use gloves, nor did he cover his hands properly. Approximately 10 days after beginning such work, his hands became extremely irritated. The irritation was itchy and seemed to produce a rash very similar to one he once had from poison ivy. He saw his physician, who prescribed a steroid cream as well as prednisone pills. He also told Phil to start wearing gloves. Phil had a good result from the medication and thought the matter was forgotten; he was certainly more careful in working with his bare hands afterward. However, about two years later, Phil's feet began to swell when he began to wear a new pair of shoes. He went to see his doctor and it was pointed out to him that the same chromate that is used in dry walls also goes into shoes. Phil had become sensitized to it during his remodeling project and the brief exposure he had by putting his feet in his shoes was enough to provoke the reaction

again. Phil could not believe it. "After all, I do wear socks," he said. However, the doctor pointed out that it only took a slight and fleeting contact for the chromate to penetrate the sock, touch his foot, and elicit the reaction. Phil thereafter displayed a healthy respect for chemicals.

For the most part, insulating materials are made of fiberglass, which has good heat and cold insulating properties. However, the small particles that are inevitably released while working with the stuff causes minor to severe skin reactions in some individuals, and the long-term effects of breathing in fiberglass fibers remain to be learned. When working with fiberglass, it is sensible to wear gloves, long sleeves, trousers that can be belted at the ankle, and a dust mask. Foam insulation made with urea formaldehyde, once popular, is now banned from use in the United States because its vapors cause a variety of quickly developing complaints such as skin and respiratory problems, headaches, as well as other more slow-to-develop reactions. If discovered during remodeling, the concentration level of its vapor should be ascertained and, if necessary, arrangements made for its removal by a firm that specializes in, and is licensed to, handle toxic materials.

Ann moved into a beautiful 1920-era pseudo-Victorian house, described by one neighbor as a monster. She was delighted with the price, but knew how much work needed to be done before it would truly be habitable. Her first step was to insulate the old monster because she knew it would cost a fortune to heat it. She hired a contractor who recommended a form of insulation made with formaldehyde. She was pleased at how easily the job was done, but the pleasure faded when she began waking up every night with a severe frontal headache. She noted that the headache never showed when she spent the night elsewhere. Finally, she read about headaches and other problems induced by the vapors of the formaldehyde used in foam insulation. She joined forces with a large group of consumers having similar complaints and after several months of complaining and facing threats of litigation, the insulation manufacturer agreed to remove the foam insulation from her house and to replace it with more benign materials.

Although foam insulation is not used anymore, there are still many thousands of homes that have it in their walls.

Roof

A roof consists of an exterior, weather-facing material (metal, plastic, ceramic tile, wood, or a mastic like tar and gravel) with an underlying moisture barrier supported by sheathing, which is ordinarily plywood or particle board resting on the rafters. As with the outside walls, insulation will underlie the sheathing.

All of the cautions we have issued about wall and floor materials also apply to the roof. The roofing material itself (especially plastics, wood shingles, or shakes treated with preservatives, fire-resistant chemicals, or the many variations of tar and gravel roofs) can release vapors that cause problems in susceptible individuals; rafters, likewise, receive preservative treatment; insulation, as already noted, carries its own threats.

Once the shell of the house is complete, the finish work begins, and this process brings a whole new series of potential allergens or irritants into the picture.

Weatherproofing Materials

At all points where doors and windows are installed, or where planes of the structure come together, or where there are joints or seams, there exist the possibility of leaks. At these points various kinds of sealants (caulking) will be interposed. These sealants are mainly soft plastics that come in a variety of colors and forms and may be applied in a number of ways. They can have pungent, irritating odors, and handling or coming in contact with them can cause rashes or irritation of the skin. When leaks do occur, asphalt carrying other chemicals and fibers will usually be applied to the site of the leak.

There are older, more traditional, safer, and, unhappily, less effective caulking materials to be had—plasters, putty, and the like. These, coupled with care given to the details of construction and appropriate use of metal flashing, can cut down materially on the use of these synthetic mastics.

Flooring

The floor itself can be made of a variety of materials—hardwoods, vinyl or other synthetic carpet materials, linoleum, ceramic tile, or concrete. Hardwoods, tile, concrete, and linoleum are relatively safe;

vinyl or other synthetic materials do present some risks. The material itself may release vapors and the adhesives used to anchor them sometimes trigger respiratory or skin problems and a host of vaguer complaints—feelings of dizziness, nausea, headaches, fatigue, malaise.

Floor coverings—carpeting in particular—can also represent a serious problem. Carpets are made from fibers, natural or synthetic. Both natural and synthetic fibers can affect sensitive individuals. Some people react to wool; cotton, even after the manufacturing process, can contain harmful residues that provoke symptoms. Grasses or other plants used to weave fiber mats can also carry contaminants; moreover, in the process of wear, they break down and the resulting microscopic fibers can be inhaled.

Synthetic carpets commonly release a formaldehyde vapor that is persistent and triggers a range of symptoms already noted. Moreover, most new synthetic carpeting is treated to make it stain-resistant. The stain-fighting chemical applied to the fiber slowly releases a gas—4-phenylcyclohexane—which, in sufficient concentration, can cause a startling array of cutaneous, vascular, and respiratory symptoms in susceptible individuals.

Carpet pads also represent a potent source of trouble. At one time such pads were made of felt or plant fibers, but lately the practice is to use polyurethane pads; these offer a nice resilient surface, but release vapors and fumes that are troublesome to those with special sensitivity to them.

The safest sort of floor is doubtless one of hardwood or ceramic tile, although it may be somewhat unforgiving to dropped dishes. However, many people make the mistake of installing a handsome hardwood floor and then protecting it with any of a variety of potentially troublesome finishes. Polyurethane is especially popular because it goes on readily, is durable, and makes a good appearance. It is worth noting, however, that the professionals who apply polyurethane wear respirator-type masks and that the fumes from it can persist and cause problems, as can those from petrochemical-based or synthetic varnishes, lacquers, or other floor finishes.

Walls and Ceiling

Sheetrock walls, once taped and textured, can receive any of a variety of finishes, almost all of which carry some risks for some individuals. Fumes from latex or acrylic-based paints cause headaches, respiratory difficulties, skin problems (rarely), and gastric upset. These finishes are easy to apply, durable, and easy to clean, but they may offgas for some period of time. Older oil-based paints can also trigger reactions and wallpapers are quite likely to be made of synthetics, to be treated with formaldehyde, and to be applied with adhesives that release persistent fumes and vapors.

The use of lead-based paints has ceased, but in some older dwellings there are still layers of lead-based paint extant. Children are particularly vulnerable to the effects of lead poisoning, which has severe behavioral and physiological consequences. If your older home has been finished with lead-based paints, seriously consider the possibility of having them removed.

In some areas of the house, particularly the recreation room or den, it is commonplace to cover the walls with "paneling" 4' x 8' x 1/4" sheets of either a very thin layer of wood veneer or wood-imitating plastics bonded to a backing, sometimes fiberboard, sometimes fine particle board. These sheets are heavily impregnated with formaldehyde resin and will offgas vapors for considerable periods of time.

The safest decorative wall and ceiling covers are untreated wood or plaster, either unfinished or covered with an essentially neutral substance like whitewash (for plaster) or a mix of boiled linseed oil and beeswax (for wood). The trouble here is that linseed oil will darken the wood to some extent; so try it out on a piece of scrap before proceeding, so that you can determine the extent to which it will darken the surface.

Heating, Plumbing, and Electrical Appliances and Fittings

Heating and air conditioning appliances are not ordinarily sources of problems, although some respiratory diseases like Legionnaires' Disease can be triggered by improperly cleaned and maintained air conditioning equipment. Heating systems that burn fossil fuels, if improperly vented or inefficient, can release gases that are troublesome or even lethal. Getting the right kind of appliances and following a careful schedule of upkeep can go a long way toward keeping the house free from allergens or irritants originating outside of or in the home. (*See* Chapter 12 for more on the selection and effective use of these devices.)

Most plumbing nowadays is plastic—polyvinyl-chloride mainly—and it can spell trouble for some people. The glues used to cement PVC pipe together are extremely pungent and the pipe itself, when new, offgasses to some extent. In addition, hot water flowing through plastic pipe causes some further offgassing and release into the water supply. Copper pipe for hot water is probably marginally preferable, although copper, too, and the lead-based solders used in its installation, does carry some slight long-term risks.

In recent years, with the cost of fossil fuels escalating, there has been a substantial move to the use of wood as a heating source. In addition to the admonition that venting should be efficient—wood smoke is a serious irritant to asthmatics and others suffering from respiratory ailments—care should be taken to minimize the added risk of fire that wood-burning heating systems represent.

Where weather conditions permit, the safest heating system is one that utilizes solar energy. There are a number of passive solar designs that have proven effective, and these represent virtually no risk to allergic or hypersensitive individuals. Finally, attention has been drawn recently to the dangers possibly presented by both the method of operation of certain electrical appliances or the electromagnetic fields they produce. Siting the house near high tension power lines may in itself be dangerous. In equipping your new house, it might pay you to be chary in your use of equipment that produces a strong electromagnetic field (microwaves, for example) or ones that generate ozone. Ozone is a particularly strong irritant, and in purchasing appliances—air conditioning or air purifying equipment for instance—the extent to which the various units under consideration produce this gas should be checked. If you manage to clean the pollen out of the air, but create a high concentration of ozone while doing so, you may find yourself no better off physically, and considerably damaged financially, for not looking closely at the manufacturer's specifications before buying.

Furnishings

The last stage of building is furnishing the new quarters, and this is where much carefully planned good work tends to be wiped out by ill-considered decisions. In general you will be well-advised to try to avoid using plastics if suitable substitutes exist. They are potent irritants, and they also represent a serious fire hazard since they burn readily and give off lethal gases when ignited. Drapes, furniture padding and coverings, shower curtains, and certain items of furniture are quite likely to be made of plastic.

New furniture, especially chests of drawers, kitchen cabinets, occasional tables, and some bed frames are increasingly being made of particle board, which, as we have already noted, consists of wood particles bonded by a urea-formaldehyde resin. These items often appeal because they are inexpensive; however, they are serious sources of irritation and they have the additional disadvantages of being ponderous and not especially durable. For a bit more money you can find unfinished pieces made of solid wood that can then be finished in ways more harmonious with your own health and esthetic needs.

Molds and Fungi

When building the new house or addition, try to take precautions as you go that will inhibit the development of the mold or fungi whose spores represent one of the more common and serious sources of allergic respiratory diseases—chronic rhinitis and asthma.

Mold and mildew thrive under damp, dark conditions, so construction strategies that will eliminate such areas should be followed. This can be accomplished by installing moisture barriers around the foundation—plastic sheets are commonly used—and by providing for adequate drainage, insuring good ventilation, installing dehumidifying equipment, being careful to seal plumbing leaks, and following a rigorous cleaning regimen that systematically monitors sources of trouble. Dark spaces under sinks, washbasins, toilet tanks, bathtubs, and shower enclosures, along window sills, and in air conditioning equipment are favorite places for mold and mildew to form. In warm, humid climates, closets can be fitted with light bulb sockets. Keeping a low wattage lightbulb burning dehumidifies the air and discourages growth of the nuisance.

Some wood used in construction is also treated with fungicides, but it is best to be careful of it because the chemicals used—dieldrin, lindane, pentachlorophenol, and tributyltin oxide—carry substantial risks for some individuals and their long-run effects are thought to be dangerous. If fungi do get established, borax or sodium carbonate can be applied; these chemicals are safe for most individuals.

A Note About Radon

Radon is a naturally occurring, colorless, odorless gas that comes from the breakdown of uranium. It is found in high concentrations in soils and rocks containing uranium, such as granite, shale, phosphate, and pitchblende. Out-of-doors it rapidly dissipates so that it does not represent a threat, but in an enclosed space like a house, it can accumulate and carries a risk of triggering cancer. It enters the house through cracks in concrete floors or cinder block walls, floor drains, plumbing entry points, and the like.

There are two measures you can take to respond to the possibility of radon contamination of your house. The first is to ascertain whether or not it exists by getting a radon detector kit and using it according to the instructions. The second thing you can do is to insure that you minimize the potential effects of the gas (if it is found to be present in significant levels) by taking care to see that you and members of your family spend as little time as possible in areas of the house showing high concentrations. In addition, whenever possible, take steps (opening windows; turning on fans) that will increase the flow of air through the dwelling. If the house has a crawl space beneath, keep all vents on all sides of the house completely open year-round. Appendix O offers procedures to follow to detect and respond to the presence of radon.

It should also be remarked that, though the level of concern about exposure to radon has been acute, most houses in the United States are not likely to suffer the problem. The scare over radon, though justified in some instances, exemplifies the American disposition to overreact to news of health aids and hazards. We would probably be much better off if the level of concern that greeted news of possible problems with radon were directed at smoking and the consumption of alcohol, which are, by many degrees, much more serious short- and long-term threats to the general health and well-being.

Points to Remember

If you or members of your family are subject to allergic or irritant reactions triggered by materials used in construction, it will pay you to investigate carefully before deciding to buy or build a home. There are literally scores of substances employed in conventional construction procedures that are capable of causing respiratory, cutaneous, or other problems, but most of them do have benign substitutes and (if you are doing the work yourself) the use of appropriate protective equipment should allow you to work safely.

Perhaps the most serious offender is formaldehyde in its various forms, partly because it is persistent, partly because it is next to impossible to manage once in place, and partly because it is very likely to be involved at all stages of construction.

Next to formaldehyde, chromate, synthetic finishes, paints, sealants, mastics, wood preservatives, polyvinylchloride, and polyurethane present the most serious potential problems to the allergic or irritant-sensitive individual. These substances, too, can be kept from use, although the main problem is that finding substitutes can be difficult, and using them in lieu of the materials commonly available will drive up the costs of construction significantly by inflating expenditures for both materials and labor.

We refer you again to Table 25, presented earlier in this chapter, which listed the major irritants or allergens encountered in the building process, details the symptoms they cause, where they are used, where they are found, and names materials that can be used in their stead.

CHAPTER 12

Inside the Home

Common Causes of Problems, the Problems They Cause, Environmental Management Devices, and Strategies for Old and New Dwellings

Home is where the heart is. Home is where we spend the bulk of our time. And home is the one place where allergens and irritants are most likely to turn up to plague us.

Combating home-based allergens or irritants successfully entails a number of steps:

- Accurately identify the allergen or irritant responsible for your symptoms
- Adopt any one or a combination of measures to avoid or control exposure in the home. These measures are:

1. Deny admission directly.
2. Erect barriers to entrance.
3. Install air cleaning devices.
4. Clean the house carefully and regularly.
5. Use hypoallergenic decor.
6. Control temperature and humidity.
7. Remove or avoid the use of triggers that are part of the structure itself.

173

Allan's asthma got worse almost immediately after his family moved into their new house. The home was only 5 years old and it had been thoroughly cleaned before they moved in. Finally, knowing the previous occupants had had cats, Allan's parents took the drastic and expensive step of tearing out and replacing all the carpets in the house. Allan got better right away.

Identify the Allergen or Irritant Responsible

Procedures to follow in establishing the cause of an allergic or toxic reaction were covered in detail in Part 3. You will remember that these procedures may:

- Help you, yourself, drawing the clear and immediate connection between symptoms and cause (noting the invariable outbreak of hives immediately after eating strawberries, for example), *or*
- Call for careful and faithful use of the allergy and irritant finders presented in Chapter 4, *or*
- Require medical consultation including a thorough physical examination followed, if necessary, by skin, laboratory, or challenge tests.

Measures to Take to Avoid or Control Exposure in the Home

Once the cause of the symptoms is confidently known, and if it is already present in the home, then the time has come to do something about it. Removing the cause, if this is possible, represents the ideal solution to allergen- or irritant-caused illness. Controlling symptoms through medication, while quite feasible for most allergic symptoms, is a decidedly second-best alternative, especially when you stop to consider the long-term costs and the possible side effects of drugs used in treatment. Here are the major tactics available to you in your effort to rid your home of allergens or irritants, or to control their appearance there.

1. Deny Admission Directly

Where the offending substance is something you can effectively interdict, simply do not allow it in the house—or if it is already there, but not part of the structure itself, cast it out. Here are some of the allergens or toxins on which this procedure is likely to be immediately and spectacularly effective:

- Animal danders (skin, saliva, or urine from furred or feathered household pets)
- Tobacco or other smoke from wood-burning stoves or fireplaces
- Household chemicals (soaps, detergents, cleaning solutions, disinfectants, insecticides)
- Fumes (candles, kerosene or gas space or water heaters or cooking stoves, adhesives, paint or other preservatives, sealants, or finishes)
- Down or feather-stuffed bedding, pillows, or apparel; other animal-based items such as wool rugs or wall hangings, feathered decor (peacock or marabou plumes), etc.

At one level the solution we suggest in each of these instances is absurdly simple—if you (or your spouse or child) is allergic to the cat, for instance, find another suitable home for the beast. If tobacco smoke causes the distress, declare the house a smoke-free zone and enforce the rule religiously; don't use household products or chemicals that cause distress—don't buy them in the first place, and if they're already in the house, give them away or throw them out; replace the wood-burning stove with electric heating appliances. Carrying out the solution, however, can be difficult. Getting rid of a pet or motivating yourself (or any other smoker in the house) to forsake the habit are tough acts. They can be done provided you are vigilant, determined, and, where applicable (quitting smoking, for example), seek out and use available help sources. Want ads are useful in finding satisfactory new homes for pets; your HMO or local Lung Association sponsors stop-smoking clinics and support groups.

2. Erect Barriers to Entrance

Where you don't lug the symptom-causing substance into the house yourself—or have the undisputed power to slam the door tightly on it—you may have to erect barriers to keep the offending substance out of the house. This tactic is appropriate for

- Plant pollens
- Outdoor dust
- Atmospheric pollutants (industrial or automotive)

Unhappily, none of these allergens is particularly easy to manage. The standard response to these invaders is to install or beef up central air conditioning. The problems are that, first, pollen- or pollutant-laden air can find ways around an air-conditioning system, especially in older, more loosely-constructed dwellings.

Second, the air conditioners themselves may not be able to remove all of the offending matter. Third, bringing in new or modifying existing systems can be expensive. Indeed, sometimes, as with rented quarters, such an approach may be out of the question.

Where central air-conditioning units are in place or installable, they can be made to work effectively by using specially made filter pads. These come in a number of different forms. First, there are extremely fine HEPA (High Efficiency Particulate Arresting) filters made of glass fibers formed into a paper-like accordion-pleated sheet. The air driven by the air conditioner fan is forced through this fine screen and it traps most of the airborne particulate material. The best of these filters will remove 99% or more of particles that are 0.3 or more microns in diameter (pollen spores measure between 8 .and 100 microns in diameter; industrial dust particles run 100 or more microns in diameter; see Figure 6 for sizes of airborne allergens or toxins). Much automotive and industrial particulate material is smaller than the 0.3 micron standard and will pass through the HEPA barrier, as will symptom-producing gases such as ozone and nitrous oxide. And to meet the 99%-removal criterion, the filter must be installed so as to make a tight seal with no blow-by. Forced air, like water, follows the path of least resistance.

HEPA filters can be quite useful, particularly for pollens, but they must be replaced periodically and this can add up to a tricky and costly business.

Central air-conditioning units can also be fitted with *"Electret"* filters, fine polyester screens that are, in effect, given an electrical charge during manufac-

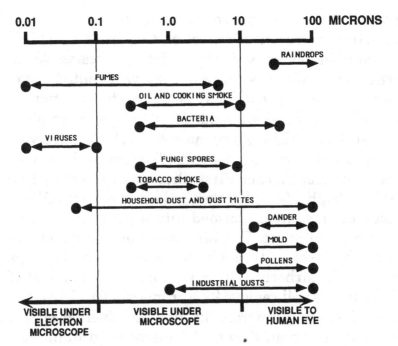

Figure 6. Size, in microns, of various airborne allergens and irritants.

ture. They act by attracting particulate matter as the air passes through the unit.

Electronic precipitators deliver an electric charge to the air as it passes through the unit. The charged particles are then attracted to polarized metal plates, much in the same way as iron filings are attracted to a magnet. Electret and precipitating-type filters need regular maintenance, either washing or (in some instances) periodic replacement.

Also available are pleated *paper filters* that do not meet HEPA standards for removal of airborne particulate material and are not particularly effective.

Appendix P lists some of the more common types of units and their more important features.

In addition to these various kinds of filters at the output side, some air-conditioners also provide for the use of pre-filters that cleanse the air before it enters the device. Pre-filters often consist of charcoal canisters and are used to remove odors and fumes.

There are a number of firms that specialize in manufacturing these various types of filters. Suppliers can be found in the Yellow Pages under "Air Conditioning Equipment and Systems Supplies and Parts — Retail," or you may want to ask the following filter manufacturers directly for price quotations and names and addresses of distributors in your locality.

E.L. Foust Inc.
Box 105
Elmhurst, IL 60126
0175 1-800-225-9549
Allergen™
electrostatic filters

Newtron Products
PO Box 27175
Cincinnati, Ohio 45277
1-800-543-9149
Self-charging
electrostatic filters

HiTech Filter Corp. of America
80 Myrtle St.
No. Quincy, MA 02171
1-800-448-3249
Self-charging electrostatic
filters

Rocky Mountain Air Inc.
3740 Paris St., Unit E
Denver, Colorado 80239
1-303-371-0272
Micretain HEPA filters

Summit Hill Laboratories
P.O. Box 535
Navesink, NJ 07552
1-800-922-0722
Micronaire electrostatic
and Hepanaire HEPA filters

As a practical matter, in the many instances where central air conditioning is either not in place or not feasible for the home, a window-mounted air conditioning unit may represent an effective alternative. Room-sized units can be fitted with any of the types of filters described above and if the device is installed snugly and the room itself is kept closed off from the rest of the dwelling it can offer the sufferer considerable relief from airborne particulate matter. Indeed, before the advent of home air conditioning, it was common practice for hay fever victims to attend an air-conditioned movie when the pollen got bad; nowadays it's off to the mall. One caution; avoid swamp coolers. Although they are extremely effective cooling units in hot, dry climates, their loosely constructed pads of wood shavings ("Excelsior") do not and are not intended to filter out airborne particles. Actually, they tend to draw pollen into the house and they frequently harbor mildew and mold that the blower fan obligingly distributes throughout the house. This is a real problem for people who live in mobile homes.

> Judy is a young immunologist. She suffers from chronic sinusitis and is very allergic to molds. It is a problem she has had all of her life, but becomes worse whenever it is damp and when she tries to cool off her home. Like many similar sufferers she has a swamp cooler in the mobile home she lives in. Her allergist is convinced that her sinusitis will improve after Judy and her husband finish building their home.

If the allergen or toxin cannot be shut out or intercepted at the door, or if it is already present in the

dwelling, you are faced with the problem of creating
and maintaining a safe interior environment. Since
at least one-third of your life is spent in bed, making
the bedroom a safe area is the most practical response.
Depending on the nature of the illness and its trigger
or triggers, you may want to consider any one or a
combination of the following measures.

3. Install Air Cleaning Devices

Room air cleaners or air purifiers (not air conditioners) are useful in controlling airborne particulate
matter, namely pollens, animal dander, molds, dust,
smoke and other pollutants (including those produced
by cooking or heating), and some gaseous material.
These devices take a number of forms but, in general,
they act by recirculating the air in the room through
some sort of collector. We encountered these collec-
tors earlier in this chapter—HEPA, Electret, or electrostatic filters, or ionizers. In essence, these units
house a fan that sucks the room air through a filter,
thus cleansing it, and then discharges it through an
outlet. There are literally dozens of these air cleaners
on the market. They range in price from under $50 to
up into the hundreds of dollars, and their effectiveness varies considerably.

Listed below are some suggestions about how to
go about selecting and using a room air cleaner.

- Be sure that you know or have a good idea about
  the exact cause of, and know the physical properties of the source of, your troubles. In particular, you will want to know the size of the offender
  and to choose equipment that will be able to trap
  it efficiently (*see* Figure 6).

- Get a unit that will circulate the air adequately. (These devices function by continually passing the air in the room through the cleansing arrangement and it will take some time—a matter of hours in fact—to remove most of the particulate matter.) For effective cleaning, the air in the room must be recycled at a rate of at least six times per hour. To find how many cubic feet of air per minute (cfm) your unit must deliver, use this equation:

Minimum cfm needed =
Room length X width X height X 6/60

For example, in a 10 by 15 ft. room with an 8-ft. ceiling, the cfm needed = 10 X 15 X 8 X 6/60 = 120.
Tabletop models are not likely to have this sort of capability.

- Some units, especially ionizing or electrostatic ones, produce ozone which is a serious irritant for susceptible individuals. Compare manufacturers' specifications for the models you are considering for purchase before making your choice. Where ozone output data are not provided, ask for them.
- Study the features of the units being compared. Determine ease, cost, and frequency of filter cleaning or replacement before buying. Dirty filters impede air flow, increase operating costs, and impair efficiency of units markedly. (The efficiency of an air purifier is ordinarily expressed as its clean air delivery rate or c.a.d.r., but this rate drops off as filters become clogged.) Also ascertain the type of fan used, whether it has variable speed options, and check it for noise. (A noisy fan may

cost you as much sleep as the other irritant.) Pay attention to weight and manageability of the unit. Some room-sized air purifiers are too heavy, bulky, and awkward to move about readily.

- Placement of the unit is an important consideration. Ideally it ought to be near the center of the room to facilitate omnidirectional recirculation of air. Finding such a central location can sometimes be a problem, and selection of a unit should be made with this difficulty in mind.
- Help the unit do its job by tightly screening windows, vents, cold air returns, and other heating cooling and ventilating arrangements with (preferably) HEPA screens. Keep doors to the room closed and use weatherproofing around door and window frames.
- Have your doctor write a prescription for the air cleaning unit and, when purchasing, be sure that the unit you select—and its accessories, like filter pads—are recognized as health measures by the US Department of Health. This makes it a deductible medical expense for tax purposes.
- If you are confused or uncertain about which product to buy, first rent a unit from a medical supply house for a trial period. Closely monitor your symptoms; if they don't improve, try another unit. Most rental firms stock a number of different makes and models.
- Compare costs, features, and effectiveness by looking at the manufacturers' technical data carefully. Consult *Consumer Reports,* which carries out and reports on periodic tests of air cleaners. The magazine's index will list the most recent article under the heading "Air Cleaners." *Con-*

sumer Reports did a complete report in the February, 1989 issue. The Association of Home Appliance Manufacturers, 20 North Wacker Drive, Chicago, IL 60606 maintains a list of certified room air cleaners. Write them for their recommendations and the specifications of the units they certify. The Allergy Products Directory (available from PO Box 640, Menlo Park, CA 94206 for $9.95) lists names and addresses of a large number of manufacturers of air cleaning devices. Some brands of air cleaners advertise features designed to counter odors, either by filtering them out or by using scent capsules to "freshen" the air. Odor-fighting filters—usually made of charcoal—aren't much more effective than good ventilation when it comes to combating odors and artificial scents trigger reactions in some susceptible individuals.

4. Clean Carefully and Regularly

Mites (*Dermatophagoides farinae*) and other foreign proteins, such as insect parts or leavings, are a major cause of respiratory disease and represent the triggering agent in what is commonly referred to as house dust allergy.

Mites are minute, free-living organisms, arthropods, members of the spider family, that subsist on human skin scales. Their inhaled leavings are a primary cause of asthma and chronic hay fever. They avoid light and require a warm, humid environment. They are persistent, prolific, and resist eradication; most insecticides that will control them are dangerous to humans. Conventional cleaning methods fail to eliminate them, either because they are found in places not efficiently reached by ordinary procedures, or the procedures themselves (vacuuming with an ordinary upright model, for example) actually disperse the organisms throughout the environment.

Air cleaners or purifiers (despite claims to the contrary) are not especially effective as a means of control of these pests because, for the most part, they are not airborne; they are best managed by careful cleaning, complemented by environmental control measures and the use of hypoallergenic decor. (*See* Sections 5 and 6 that follow.)

The area to be cleaned—usually the bedroom— should feature clear, smooth surfaces to the fullest possible extent. These surfaces should be mopped every two to three days with a clean damp cloth. If the person who does the cleaning is also the one who reacts to dust, he or she should wear a mask capable of filtering out particles one micron in diameter. Ordinary paper masks of the kind worn by construction workers will not meet this standard; see the Allergy Products Handbook referred to above for the names of suppliers of more efficient masks. However, if you have asthma, be very careful about wearing any special restrictive mask.

> Liz, a laboratory technician, is very sensitive to the smell of formaldehyde, which aggravates her asthma. Because of this she bought a tight fitting mask called a Wilson II; it is a great protective device but it also reduces Liz's the air intake. Accordingly, Liz has to breathe harder when she wears it and this hyperventilation makes her asthma worse.

Table 26
Avoiding Household Dust

General Household	Bedrooms
Avoid home furnishings that are likely to capture dust • fabric wall hangings, tapestries • stuffed animals • upholstered or ornately carved furniture	Remove all potential dust collecting articles • carpeting • wall decorations • books etc.
Keep dust-gathering places clean • radiators and heating vents • pay attention to home appliances, e.g., TVs and stereos	Use a HEPA or other air purification system; use air conditioning • control dust mites by keeping humidity below 50%
Use easy to clean, hard finish surfacing materials e.g., bare wood, fiberglass, metal, plastics	Use plastic or plain wood furnishings • replace window treatments (drapes, curtains, etc.) with roll down window shades
Clean regularly with damp mop and sponge (every other day, if possible) If vacuuming is necessary, use a tank or canister type	Clean frequently • wash blankets every 2–4 weeks • damp mop floors regularly (every other day if possible) • dust drawers, closets, etc. regularly
	Store clothing in a cleaned, closed closet
	Use synthetic or cotton bed linens • avoid products containing down, feathers, or wool
	Avoid stuffed animals • if not possible, provide washable or easily cleaned stuffed toys

Table 27
Sites for Allergens or Irritants Inside the Home

Site	Response	Replacement
Carpets, rugs	Discard	None
Fabric wall hangings	Discard	None
Plush dolls; stuffed toys	Discard	Appropriate dust-free toys
Upholstered furniture	Discard	Plain wood or plastic pieces
Fabric drapes	Discard	Plastic drapes, pull down blinds; slatted, easy-to-clean blinds
Fabric bed headboard	Discard	Plain wood or plastic covered
Bedspread	Discard	None
Books and magazines	Keep to minimum	Store in closed book-case. Dust regularly
Electronic gear	See preceding section	
Forced air heating systems	Close off heating vents	Install electric or radiant heating
Air conditioning vents	Cover tightly with HEPA or electrostatic air filters	
Mattress, box spring, pillows	Encase in plastic covers	
Wool blankets, down or feather pillows or comforters	Discard	Cotton blankets, fiberfill or synthetics
Clothing	Keep picked up. Store soiled clothes in plastic bags, clean clothes in plain wooden chest of drawers or closet. Keep wool clothing encased in plastic garment bags. *Do not* use camphor or other moth or insect repellents.	

In addition to regular, thorough, attentive dust-mopping of all surfaces, dust-attracting devices should receive special attention. Electronic gear—radios, TVs, hi-fis, speakers, VCRs, computers, etc.—should be kept as free as possible of dust, stored in an enclosed space, and covered when not in use. House plants also catch dust (as well as generate mold, mildew, and plant spores or pollen) and should be relegated to the guest room. Venetian or similar slatted blinds should be gone over carefully on each cleaning occasion. Table 26 illustrates an approach to keeping your home dust free. Special cleaning or polishing agents are not necessary and, in fact, some of them are known to trigger reactions in some persons. The major home of dust and dust mites is the bed itself. Bedding (sheets, pillow cases, blankets) should be changed and washed at least once weekly in water at a temperature of 70 or more degrees centigrade (145 degrees Fahrenheit). Several firms manufacture special vacuum cleaners that feature either water traps, HEPA filters, or high suction. These devices have not been sufficiently studied to establish their efficacy and their price ($500–$800) makes us cautious about recommending them as an adjunct to the considerably lower-tech cleaning procedures recommended above.

5. Use Hypoallergenic Decor

Hypoallergenic decor—furnishing, decorating, and equipping the room with furniture and accessories that do not provide a haven for dust, mites, pollen, danders, or other reaction-producing substances—often proves helpful. Tables 26 and 27 show you how you can deal with some common havens for problems.

Of all the measures listed in Table 27, the most effective single one is likely to be the one recommending use of plastic covers on mattress, box spring, and pillows. Local suppliers may be found under Medical Equipment and Supplies in the Yellow Pages; the Allergy Products Directory, mentioned above, also lists vendors of bedding supplies, and a few suppliers are named in Appendix Q.

6. *Control Temperature and Humidity*

Controlling temperature and humidity may put you in something of a Catch-22 situation. If you have asthma, your symptoms are liable to be less severe in a warmer, moister environment. Unhappily, mites also thrive under these conditions. Thus, if your asthma can be traced to dust mites, what helps you also helps them.

Molds and mildew represent a significant cause of respiratory problems; they, too, thrive under moist conditions, and they can be found almost anywhere. Maintaining a temperature of 22 degrees Celsius (70 degrees Fahrenheit) or more and relative humidity of 50% or less will help to combat mites and mold, although both of these triggers are stubborn, year-round problems that demand constant attention. Insofar as the interior of the house is concerned, Table 28 lists some of the places that mold and mildew are likely to be encountered and the measures you can take to combat them.

A special word should be said about humidifiers or vaporizers. These are devices sold at most drug stores that are commonly used to help children with croupy coughs. They consist of a basin, filled with

Table 28
Locations of and Measures to Control Mold
and Mildew in and Around the Home

Site	Countermeasure
Bedroom	
Mattress or box springs	Encase in plastic coverings
Closets	Use low watt electric bulb as heat and drying source; put out hygroscopic crystals, available at your local drugstore, to absorb moisture. *Caution! Hygroscopic Crystals Are Poisonous If Ingested and Should Be Kept Away from Children*
Bathroom	
Damp areas under sinks, around toilets, bathtubs, toilet tanks, showers, soap dishes, shower curtains, tile, bath mats, clothes hampers, window sills	Clean carefully with solutions of liquid bleach, Pine Sol, or Lysol
Living Areas	
Potted plants	Move or discard
Aquariums	Move or discard
Walls	Clean with solution as above. If wall remains damp, seal with moisture sealer or barrier and refinish if necessary
Windowsills	Clean with solution as above
Fireplace	Clean with solution as above. Keep flues closed when not in use. Seal exterior to provide water and vapor barrier
Heating or air conditioning units or vents	Mask with HEPA or other screen
Vaporizers and humidifiers	Clean frequently with solution as above to kill mold and mildew
Kitchen	
Under sinks, window sills, refrigerator coils, dishwashers	Clean with solution as above
Food in pantries, bins, breadboxes, etc.	Discard spoiled food; clean containers or receptacles carefully, dry thoroughly
Garage and Basement	
Water heater	Repair any leaks. Clean with solution as above
Garbage cans	Clean with solution regularly
Wet footwear, clothes, or rags	Clean or wash, as appropriate, and dry thoroughly
Wet garden hoses	Drain after use, dry, coil or store on reel
Pet litter boxes	Empty regularly and clean with solution
Exterior Landscaping	Keep hedges and lawn trimmed, clean up piles of leaves, cuttings, and compost. Avoid creating wet spots if irrigating

water, and a fan that vaporizes the water. The basins often are invaded by mold and can cause pneumonia and make asthma worse. It is very important therefore that they be regularly cleaned with vinegar to kill the mold.

7. Remove or Avoid Using Triggers That Are an Integral Part of the Structure Itself

A substantial number of the materials used in or produced as a byproduct of the construction, maintenance, or operation of buildings are capable of triggering reactions in vulnerable persons. Table 25 in the preceding chapter lists some of the more important offenders, where they are found, and the reactions they may provoke, and suggests appropriate counter measures.

Detecting and controlling these reaction-causing in-house substances is often a difficult matter. For one thing, the symptoms are likely to be subacute, attributable to any of a legion of other possible causes. Vague feelings of malaise, intermittent headaches, fleeting giddiness or disorientation, or chronic fatigue can be charged up to infections, stress, or any of a host of other conditions. This often makes drawing a clear connection between cause and symptom complicated and uncertain.

Secondly, in the absence of appropriate and readily available tests, the offender is often next to impossible to single out, and even if it is detected it may be virtually impossible to do anything about it. For instance, if formaldehyde originating in particleboard subflooring is responsible for your distress, you have very few options and they are, at the least, bound to be expensive, and disruptive.

If you suspect that something in your home or some part of the structure itself—is causing your symptoms, make the best possible record you can—when, where, how often, and under what circumstances they occur, what they are, and how they affect you. Then take your analysis to an allergist who is interested in and has knowledge of and experience in environmentally caused toxic or allergic reactions. Table 25 can be used as a rough guide to the more common kinds of reactions to materials used in constructing dwellings. The allergy department of a teaching hospital or university medical school is probably the best source of the specialized kind of help that may be required to nail down the cause of house-borne symptoms and to develop effective measures to counter them.

Points to Remember

This chapter provides a series of strategies that are designed to help you get allergens or irritants out of your house—and your life.

The task is by no means easy—it requires careful planning, scrupulous attention to detail, and unrelenting follow through. Controlling allergens and irritants is a difficult and tedious job. Knowing what to do and how to go about doing it—the message here—will make the job much easier, more systematic, and more understandable. Following the procedures we have outlined will save you time, money, grief—as well as the discomfort and suffering that allergen or irritant-triggered diseases cause.

CHAPTER 13

At Work

*Substances and Technologies Causing Problems
and How to Avoid Their Effects*

The relationship of ill health to working conditions has been known for nearly 300 years. A famous
publication by the Italian physician, Bernardo
Ramazzini, in the year 1713, first drew attention to
diseases associated with specific occupations when it
pointed out the increased prevalence of asthma and
other respiratory complaints among bakers. Although
bakers' asthma is of historical importance because it
was the initial connection of occupation to disease, the
list of such conditions and diseases has grown to considerable length and keeps expanding as new classes
of chemicals crowd into the workplace.

Occupationally Linked Diseases
of the Airways

Airway diseases associated with work are usually
divided into those that affect the nose and sinuses
(upper airways) and those that involve the lungs (lower airways). The agents that provoke the symptoms
and the industries in which they are encountered
make a formidably long list. The occupations and the

Table 29
Occupations or Industries in Which Allergic Upper
or Lower Airway Disease Occurs,
and the Agents Known to Provoke the Symptoms

Occupation or industry	Agent
Aluminum solderer	Aminoethyl ethanolamine (flux)
Animal handlers	Animal products
Automobile spray painters	Hexamethylene diisocyanate
Bakers/millers	Wheat/rye/buckwheat flour, fungal amylase (enzyme)
Bird fanciers	Birds (Budgerigars)
Brewery chemist/worker	Hops, sulfone chloramides
Cabinet maker/carpenter/ construction, wood, or sawmill workers	Wood dust (California Red cedar, redwood, oak, mahogany)
Chemist	Piperazine chloride (drug)
Crab processor	Crab
Detergent industry worker	*B. subtilis* (enzyme)
Electronics	Colophony (flux)
Entomologists	Moths, butterflies
Epoxy resins, plastics	Phthalic, trimelletic, or tetrachlorophthalic anhydrides
Fish bait breeder	Bee moth
Flight crews	Screw worm fly
Food processor	Coffee beans
Foundries	Diphenyl diisocyanate
Foundry mold making	Furfuryl, alcohol
Grain workers/handlers	Grain mite, grain dust
Gum manufacturing	Gum tragacanth
Hairdresser	Persulfate salts, henna
Hard metal industry	Cobalt, vanadium, tungsten, carbide
Hospital staff	Hexachlorophene (sterilizing agent), formalin
Insulation/resin manu- facturing or handling	Urea, formaldehyde
Laboratory workers	Rats, mice, guinea pigs, rabbits, cockroaches, papain (enzyme)
Laxative manufacturing	Psyllium

(continued...)

Table 29 *(continued)*

Occupation or industry	Agent
Metal plating	Nickel
Food oil industry	Castor bean
Oyster farming, processing	Hoya
Packaging	Papain (enzyme)
Pharmaceutical	Enzyme, trypsin, pancreatin, pepsin, flaviastase, bromelain, toluene diisocyanate, penicillins, cephalosporin, phenylglycine acid chloride, methyl dopa, spiramycin, salbutamol intermediate, tetracycline
Photocopying and dying	Diazonium salt
Photography	Ethylene diamine
Plastics/rubber	Trypsin (enzyme), azodicarbonamide
Platinum refining	Platinum
Polyurethane	Toluene diisocyanate
Poultry workers	Chicken
Prawn processing	Prawn
Printer	Gum acacia
Refrigeration	Freon
Sericulture	Larva of silkworm
Spray painter	Dimethyl ethanolamine
Tanning	Chromium
Tea worker	Tea
Tobacco manufacturing	Tobacco leaf
Veterinarian	Animal danders (all)

triggers that have been linked in the medical litera-
ture with allergic respiratory disease are named in
Table 29.

Beyond the substances named in Table 29, all of
which have been cited in medical reports as provoking airway disease, there are a number of other occupations or conditions of work that have long been tied

to respiratory symptoms. Smoke, dust, or airborne particles are well-established as triggers, as are vapors from paints or varnishes, especially those containing volatile organic compounds or urethanes. Fumes from adhesives or glues, heating or cooking gas, fluxes used in soldering or welding, lint, animal dander, or insect parts can all cause asthma, rhinitis, and other forms of respiratory distress in susceptible individuals, and they can affect anyone from acupuncturist to zoologist. Even people in the most benign-appearing jobs may wind up sick.

> Reg had asthma as a child, but the symptoms gradually faded away as he matured. He had no recurrence until he was in his forties and accepted an invitation to be a visiting professor at an African university. The University supplied housing for its staff and, soon after moving into his new quarters, Reg's asthma returned with a vengeance. He and the University physician finally figured out that he was severely allergic to the cashew trees that surrounded his house—the University had been built on the site of a cashew plantation and the trees were spared. Reg's symptoms were so persistent and severe that he had to return to his university where, interestingly enough, he started showing mild asthmatic symptoms to tree pollens there.

It is surprisingly difficult to establish a diagnosis of occupation-associated respiratory disease. If the symptoms turned up only when the worker was at the job, the connection would be transparently clear. Unhappily for the diagnostician and the sufferer there are delayed as well as immediate reactions. For example, if you are allergic to the sting of a bee you will develop symptoms as soon as you are stung; someone allergic to penicillin will show a reaction immediately upon ingestion of, or being injected with, this antibiotic. However, in the case of occupation-associated allergies, the reactions may be delayed for considerable periods of time.

> Bert works in the plastic industry. He is fine when he is at work, but virtually every night about 11:00 PM or midnight he wakes up with severe wheezing. The wheezing persists for several hours and is nearly always gone by the next morning. At first he thinks something at home is causing his problem; he has had it for several months and did not associate it with anything at work until he took a vacation. Then, almost immediately, his nocturnal wheezing stopped, even though he spent the entire vacation at home. He discussed this with his doctor, who quickly determined that Bert was allergic to some of the plastic fumes he was exposed to at work.

Specific skin tests and sometimes even inhalation challenge tests can be administered to help diagnose the cause when occupational respiratory allergies are suspected. Challenge tests, the most dependable way, attempt to recreate what actually occurs in the workplace. Thus, if you are thought to be reacting to plastic fumes, your physician may have you inhale a solution of the same plastic fumes you encounter at work. However, such a challenge can be dangerous—even life threatening—and should only be done in cases where the diagnosis is unclear or the condition is such that significant disability will occur unless an accurate diagnosis is established. And it should be done only under careful medical supervision with a full array of emergency materials and devices on hand and immediately available.

It has been said that the best physicians rely most heavily on the stethoscope and what lies between the ear pieces. We certainly subscribe to this judgment, believing that the medical interview is the most important element in diagnosing occupational illness. The specific factors taken into account should include an inventory of all materials found in the workplace, information on air exchange within the space, and medical histories of other personnel who work in the area. It should look for obviously correlated respiratory problems, including a history of tobacco smoking.

The Federal Occupational Safety and Health Administration (OSHA) has taken an active role in preventing occupation-associated respiratory disease, and standards have been established for workers employed in specific industries. Workers exposed to toluene diisocyanate have been objects of special concern; careful monitoring and surveillance of individuals and the workplace is required in industries using this compound. However, in many industries idiosyncratic reactions may occur that are not easily explained.

> John works in a dry-milk processing plant in Wisconsin. He is a life-long asthmatic with allergies rampant in his family. Thus, his doctor was not surprised when John's asthma became more difficult to treat. However, he became suspicious when he learned that the asthma seemed to improve whenever John took a trip. The Doctor checked further and learned that in manufacturing milk powder the process resulted in the milk occasionally becoming an aerosol. John, in inhaling it, developed a localized, milk-induced asthma.

Another form of work-related respiratory disease is the one that results when airborne material develops during the manufacturing process. For example, a variety of enzymes are used in the pharmaceutical or food processing industries. These enzymes include papain, chymopapain, and bromelain. When used in large quantities and subjected to heat, they may develop into an aerosol—minute particles suspended in the air—and become a part of the air you breathe on the job. Exposure to even a tiny quantity of these agents is often enough to trigger an allergic reaction.

In addition to the materials that are used in manufacturing or processing products, there are other allergens or irritants that inhabit working areas. Mold is by far the most common of these resident triggers. Mold is not just something you find under your bathroom sink in the winter. Rather, it is a common problem anywhere there is moisture. It is likely to be found in any situation that uses water in the manufacturing process or in excessively damp or moist environments—chemical plants, dairies, food processing plants, farms, silos, grain storage elevators, or even in faulty air conditioners. Thus, occupational respiratory disease may result not only from the materials that are part of the manufacturing process, but from the working conditions themselves—moist, dusty, poorly ventilated, excessively hot or cold environments. Tactics for controlling or eliminating noxious respiratory agents so that the workplace is made safe for you should include

- Installing engineering refinements that either eliminate the trigger entirely or (through the introduction of hoods, exhaust fans, traps, filters, or other air-cleansing devices) minimize contact with it.

- providing protective respiratory devices—any of several kinds of masks designed to protect you from harmful particles and fumes.
- maintaining work areas at an acceptable level of cleanliness.
- improving surveillance of the overall conditions of work, perhaps through employer–employee agreement and cooperation.
- enforcing compliance with health and safety precautions strictly and vigorously.
- where necessary, and under circumstances in which other measures for the control of allergens or irritants fail, moving you to a job or work site that is free of the irritants.

All of these measures assume some disposition on the part of the employer to take corrective action with the physical well-being of you, the employee, held paramount. Unhappily, in our experience all too many employers fail to recognize that the health of their employees is reflected importantly in the health of their own profit and loss statements. They take little or no action to rectify unsafe or unhealthy working conditions. If this happens to be the case with your employer, you do have recourse and the actions open to you are spelled out in Part 6.

Occupationally Linked Skin Diseases

There are literally thousands of substances in the workplace that are capable of causing skin reactions.

Whether or not they do trigger symptoms in you depends on two factors—your degree of atopy and the
level of exposure you are subjected to.

We dealt with the concept of atopy in Chapter 2.
Atopic individuals, we noted, are genetically susceptible to allergic reactions, even from casual exposure
to triggers. But, even people who are not atopic and
have no history of allergic disease can develop symptoms if the level or duration of exposure is high
enough.

To illustrate the effect of chronic, intense exposure to an allergen/irritant, some years ago an experiment was carried out on 20 rural Kentuckians. They
had been in frequent and direct contact with poison
ivy all of their lives and none of them had ever developed poison ivy symptoms. They were asked essentially to bathe in poison ivy. With this high degree of
exposure, eventually every one of the volunteers did
develop sensitivity—and probably lived to regret vol-
unteering to participate in that particular experiment.

Skin allergies or irritations account for a substantial majority of compensation awards for industrial
disease. It is believed that the actual prevalence of
contact dermatitis in the workplace is significantly
underestimated and underreported.

Occupationally linked skin diseases include hives
(urticaria), redness or inflammation (erythema), and
flushing (transient erythema), accompanied by local-
ized swelling, pain, intense itching (pruritus), the development of rashes, blisters or vesicles, and cracking of the skin. Table 30 lists some of the occupations
or industries commonly associated with cutaneous
reactions and the agents that cause them.

Table 30
Occupations or Industries in Which Contact
Dermatitis Occurs, and the Agents Known
to Provoke the Symptoms

Agent*	Occupation or industry
Chromate	Construction workers (cement finishers, wallboard tapers/ texturers), engineering trades (workers exposed to metals and soluble oils containing chromate), tanners, milk testers, printers, printing plate makers
Nickel	Occupations involving exposure to coinage, nickel-plated instruments, and soluble oils containing nickel; metal workers, machinists, construction workers, metal polishers
Cobalt	Occupations involving production of hard metal; electrical and electronic workers; persons involved in the manufacture or use of some paints and varnishes
Thiourams and mercaptobenzothiazole (MBT)	Mainly in occupations requiring use of rubber gloves or other rubber apparel as protective equipment (surgeons, nurses, dentists, dental assistants) or needed in "wet" work (cleaners, gardeners, housewives)
Paraphenylenediamine (PPD)	Individuals using PPD dyes in hairdressing; individuals handling industrial rubber
Resin	Ubiquitous; found in sizing in clothes, coatings on paper products, printing inks, cutting oils, flux (for solder)

(continued...)

Table 30 *(continued)*

Agent*	Occupation or Industry
Formaldehyde	Occupations involving manufacture of formaldehyde or products containing it; building trades workers, textile workers, furriers, leather workers, health care providers, pathologists, morticians
Epoxy resins	Electrical industry (manufacturing of circuit boards, cathodic insulation installers); industries using fiberglass (aircraft, automobile, marine, furniture)

*The agents listed in this table are the more common and important ones; it makes no claim to being exhaustive.

Claude's hobby is building fishing rods. He noted that a while after he started working on graphite models—the latest wonder material—his hands, forearms, and eyelids broke out in a stubborn rash. He went to his doctor, and was sent on to a dermatologist who established that Claude's skin problems were dermatitis caused by the epoxy resin used to coat the windings.

The cause of an occupationally caused skin disease is usually apparent and the tactics for controlling or dealing with it are the same as the ones listed earlier in this chapter in connection with work-related airway disease.

A Note About Workers' Compensation

In general, job-related injuries or illnesses are covered by insurance that employers are required to carry on their employees. In Chapter 17 we've sketched the steps you can take to invoke this protection, which provides for medical treatment and compensation during any period of job-related disability. If you are made ill through no fault of your own, by conditions or materials that you encounter on the job, you are entitled to this sort of care and support and should seek it out aggressively and without being made to feel as if your were disloyal or malingering.

Points to Remember

Work-related allergies or hypersensitivities are commonplace and likely to be underreported. There are legions of substances found in the workplace that are capable of triggering respiratory or skin problems, the usual sites of occupational allergies. Probably no job (or worker) is entirely free or safe from threat.

In most instances the risk posed by these substances can be reduced by ridding the working environment of the hazard or using appropriate protective gear. Although a few of the substances can cause chronic symptoms, eliminating or avoiding them is usually followed quickly by a complete recovery with no complications.

CHAPTER 14
In Health Care Settings

It's reasonable to think that the doctor's or dentist's office, the hospital, or the health clinic ought to be a safe place, relatively free of allergens or toxins. Think again!

Esperanza, 9, is in the allergy clinic with her mother to get her monthly hay fever booster shot. The nurse pulls her chart, checks on the strength of medication required, prepares the required dose. She calls Esperanza into the consulting room, swabs the child's arm with alcohol, and administers the dose. The child returns to the waiting room to let the required 30 minutes pass. She tells her mother that she is thirsty and asks permission to go down the hall for a drink of water. Mother says, "Go ahead." Esperanza gets up and goes out. After a few minutes the mother becomes concerned that the child has not returned and goes to the drinking fountain. She sees a number of people huddled around a form lying on the floor. It is Esperanza, and the personnel from another department are administering mouth-to-mouth resuscitation in what ultimately proves to be a vain attempt to return the child to consciousness. An hour later Esperanza is declared dead. Mishaps like Esperanza's are not uncommon. The strength of the dose of antigen that the nurse injected was too great for the child. She had slipped into shock and by the time help had reached her, it was too late.

205

Reaction to the administration of allergy shots is the most common cause of anaphylaxis or shock, and each year a substantial number of people die after receiving an allergy shot. Sometimes human error is at fault; more often, though, it is the unavoidable result of unexpected and unforeseeable hypersensitivity of the patient to the medication being administered.

Here are the major causes of serious hypersensitive reactions in health care settings:

1. Injections of antigens to desensitize individuals to allergens, mainly the ones responsible for hay fever symptoms.
2. Injections of other drugs that trigger severe reactions.
3. Reactions to medications taken orally or topically.
4. Exposure to processes or substances in the health care setting itself, either part of or incidental to the treatment regimen, that are capable of causing illness or injury.

Each of these possible sources of illness or injury and the steps that you or your health care provider can take in order to avoid or minimize them are spelled out in the sections that follow.

Allergy Shots

A common and time-honored method of treatment of some allergic symptoms is to desensitize the individual to whatever it is that is causing the problem. This procedure works fairly well for many hay fever sufferers, and for people who react seriously to stings of hymenoptera (honey bees and other members of that family) and bites of triatoma (assassin or kissing bugs). It works less well and can be particularly dangerous for asthmatics. Allergy shots are contraindicated for eczema, hives, and nearly all allergic skin diseases.

The use of allergy shots depends, first, on determining exactly what is causing your symptoms by administering skin (scratch or prick) tests and then injecting you with a very mild concentration of the substance found to cause the problem. If you are diagnosed as being allergic to grass pollens, for instance, the desensitization procedure would have you coming into the allergist's office every week or two where you would get, at first, an injection of an extremely dilute solution of the pollen causing your distress. The concentration of the substance being injected would gradually be increased over time until your body would not respond to the equivalent of a dose ordinarily capable of provoking the undesirable hay fever symptoms. (The procedure simply uses a nicely graduated series of doses to lead—some might even say "trick"— the body into developing a lack of sensitivity to the invader.)

As we have seen in the case of Esperanza, this procedure carries risks. There is always the possibility of human error, the chance that too-strong a dose will be prepared and administered with unpleasant or even lethal consequences. In addition to human error, there are other factors that can produce serious reactions. In some instances when symptoms are already present, but not readily apparent or sub-threshold, the antigen, even if properly formulated, can add to the existing level of sensitivity—this is called a synergistic response—and trigger symptoms. In other instances, the administration of an antigen can bring on symptoms that are part of the constellation of allergic diseases, although not the ones originally prompting the treatment. Hay fever shots can and do trigger asthma or skin diseases like eczema or hives in some susceptible individuals. In others whose immunological systems are in some way compromised, allergy shots can make the disease worse. Thus, we do not recommend allergy shots for people with diabetes, lupus, rheumatoid arthritis, or any so-called autoimmune disease. We also do not recommend allergy shots for individuals with AIDS or who test positive for HIV.

There is another problem with allergy shots. The potency of the antigens used as the basis for preparing the dose vary considerably, both from vendor to vendor and, over time, from the same vendor. Even with the most careful and demanding of procedures, you can never be sure of the potency of what is being jabbed into you. Your health care provider can partially guard against this by sticking to the practice of buying from laboratories that make strong efforts to standardize their products for consistency and potency, but this stricture is often violated. In addition you may move or your child may go off to college and be given a different batch from a new doctor.

Here are suggestions on how to avoid the risk of allergic or hypersensitive reactions when undergoing desensitization.

1. Avoid skin or scratch testing for sensitivity to given kinds of allergens if you are showing any asthmatic symptoms at all. (If you are already sneez-

ing or wheezing from pollen, scratch- or prick-skin testing would likely be useless for diagnostic purposes and would carry the risk of intensifying whatever symptoms you are already showing.)

2. If you have eczema, absolutely avoid skin testing, since it may aggravate your symptoms. (*See* Chapter 9 for an alternative to skin testing.)

3. If desensitization is in order (and it is in order much less often than it is prescribed; shots for asthma or stomach disorders resulting from food hypersensitivity are rarely appropriate, for example) be sure that there are patient safeguards in place. There should be at least a 30-minute, closely monitored waiting period after the injection is given. There should be people immediately on hand who have been trained in, know, and can carry out emergency procedures. There should be necessary first aid supplies (epinephrine; antihistamines) instantly available, and there should be a physician present or summonable on immediate notice. In addition, when the post-injection waiting period is completed, there should be a careful inspection of the patient by whoever made the injection to note and record the magnitude of the reaction, if any, and other associated signs such as swelling, itchiness at the site, general itchiness, hives, pallor, difficulty in breathing, faintness, dizziness. If any of these symptoms does show up, the patient should be watched carefully and not permitted to leave until they have abated because any of these signs suggest the person may be at risk.

4. If, after diagnosis, a course of allergy shots is recommended, invest in a second opinion. Ask

your family doctor, internist, or pediatrician for suggestions. A fair number of allergists have "needle" practices in which their main tactic is to get and maintain a cadre of patients coming in for weekly, semiweekly, or monthly shots. For these practitioners, it may be more important to recruit a steady supply of arm-baring patients than to prescribe alternative methods of treatment that are both cheaper and at least as effective as getting on the shots treadmill.

5. If you are having allergy shots, make sure they are being given by Board-certified allergist, and not by an Ear-Nose-Throat, or any other, specialist. The only medical specialists who receive training in the proper choice and routine administration of allergy shots are allergists. *See* Chapter 17 on choosing a doctor.

Ms. Jackson was disappointed that her doctor was retiring. She had been seeing him for over 30 years and every Monday, without fail, she had reported at his office to get her allergy shot. She had long forgotten what she was supposed to be allergic to. Her doctor, though, gave her the large brown bottle that had appeared for each shot session and advised her to see someone at the medical center nearby. Her new doctor, who was also an allergy professor at the medical school, took the bottle Ms. Jackson had brought to him at their first meeting. He couldn't believe what he saw. Ms. Jackson had received 30 years' worth of shots from a bottle labeled "Ms. Jackson's Potion." Whatever was in the bottle originally must have long been rendered ineffective by age and deterioration.

Reactions to Injections

Apart from getting allergy shots, there are three other commonplace reasons for being injected:

- To receive medication for some sort of infection
- To be anesthetized
- To be immunized against certain diseases

Each of these routine encounters with the syringe can offer a risk to the susceptible person.

Infections

One of the major medical advances of the past half-century has been the discovery of a multitude of drugs with the ability to attack infections—mainly bacterial infections—directly. Prior to the advent of these "wonder drugs"—antibiotics for the most part— a physician was pretty much limited to trying to relieve the symptoms while the body set about mending itself. With the appearance of drugs like sulfa, penicillin, tetracycline, and so on, it became possible for the doctor to address the organism directly responsible for the symptoms.

Most of these new drugs can be given to the patient in a number of ways, but administering a "shot," especially to deliver a significant amount of medication rapidly, remains a routine aspect of treatment for some physicians. Yet, almost always there are drugs that, when given orally, are just as effective and much less risky for the recipient.

We have listed some of the commonly used injectable antibiotics known to trigger allergic or hypersen-

Table 31
Antibiotic Triggers, Their Trade Names,
the Conditions for Which They Are Prescribed,
and the Reactions They Are Known to Provoke

Antibiotic	Trade names	Prescribed for	Reactions
Penicillin	Penicillin, Ampicillin, Amoxicillin Augmentin, dozens of other names	Strep throat, pneumonia, sinuses, ear and urinary tract infections	Rash, hives anaphylaxis
Sulfonamides	Gantrisin Bactrim	Ear and urinary tract infections	Rash, hives serum sickness, anaphylaxis
Cephalosporins	Kefzol, Ceftin	Strep throat, pneumonia, sinusitis	Rash, hives, anaphylaxis
Erythromycin	Too many to list	Strep throat, pneumonia	Severe gastritis, occasionally jaundice
Tetracyclines	Minocin Terramycin	Acne, diarrhea respiratory infections, UTIs	Teeth turn yellow, rashes

sitive reactions in Table 31. Also presented are the trade names under which the drug is sold, the conditions for which it is likely to be administered, and the kinds of reactions or side effects it may trigger. (It is obviously impracticable in a general book of this kind to specify all of the antibiotics and the complaints at which they can be aimed, so the list is meant to be illustrative rather than complete.)

Since the administration of an injectable drug will be carried out in the healthcare-provider's office or the clinic, it is important for you to find out exactly what is to be administered, the strength of the dose, and its possible side effects. The doctor or technician should supply this information routinely; if this is not done, demand that the information be given to you before submitting to the needle. If you know that you react to any drugs, be sure that you convey this information to the care provider beforehand. Finally, where drugs are being given that carry the risk of precipitating an anaphylactic or "shock" reaction, (penicillin is a particularly likely trigger) the countermeasures and precautions listed earlier in this chapter in connection with allergy shots should be in place. Most important, ask your doctor whether you couldn't just take a pill instead of being injected; and, if not, why not.

Sarah will never forget the day she saw her doctor for a sore throat that was raw and painful and accompanied by a fever. Her doctor said she had strep throat and decided to give her a shot of long-acting penicillin—procaine penicillin. Sarah anticipated no problems; she had often had penicillin in the past. However, within minutes of receiving the shot she developed hives all over her body; then she began gasping for breath. The doctor had to give her two shots of adrenalin, hook her up to an IV to administer fluids, and admit her to the hospital overnight. Sarah probably did need the penicillin, but her anaphylactic reaction would likely not have occurred if she had been given pills instead of a shot.

Table 32
Injectable Anesthetics Causing Reactions, When and
Why They Are Used, and the Side Effects They Cause

Anesthetic	When/why used	Side reactions
Novocaine	Routine dental extractions	Rash, anaphylaxis
Xylocaine	Local surgery	Rash, anaphylaxis
Citanest	Local surgery	Rash, anaphylaxis
Procaine/ procainamide	Dentistry; local surgery	Rash, anaphylaxis

Anesthetics

Though the dentist is the health care provider most likely to administer an anesthetic, almost everyone at one time or another will experience a medical problem that will call for the injection of a local or general anesthetic. Table 32 lists the injectable anesthetics in common use, when and why they are likely to be required, and the sorts of undesirable side effects they are capable of producing in the susceptible individual.

When you know that you react adversely to a particular anesthetic, be sure to remind the person who will administer it that you do have a problem. And, as a matter of practice, try wherever possible to undergo the procedure without the aid of anesthetics. This is particularly true in dental care, where much of the anesthetizing is done for the dentist's, rather than the patient's, benefit. Using an anesthetic makes it possible for the dentist to devote much less time to the patient. Yet, many superficial dental procedures can be carried out by adopting a more leisurely pace of treatment coupled with the use of benign, but more time-consuming procedures such as cold applications, masking sound, and the like. You are entitled to have your wishes heard and, wherever possible, acceded to; you are more than an interchangeable part on a dental assembly line, drugged to the point at which you can be dealt with roughly in the shortest possible unit of time so that the dentist can scurry down the hall to the next patient while you take hours to recover from the numbness he or she leaves behind.

> Lisa was a lovely teenager. She had an impacted wisdom tooth that needed extracting. Her parents, new in town, picked a dentist by reading a newspaper ad. The dentist, pushed for time, so he said, told the mother that, to speed things along, he'd give her a little dose of harmless laughing gas. Lisa made the papers the next morning. She had died from an overdose of the gas. Her dentist was eventually arrested for manslaughter; it turned out that Lisa was the *third* patient fatality that had occurred in his office—all from gas overdose.

Immunization

Inoculating children and adults to confer immunity to common infectious diseases is a routine medical procedure. Although there are reports, each year, of a few severe-to-fatal reactions to these vaccines, their benefits far outweigh their risks. Nevertheless, some individuals are extremely susceptible to these procedures and the decision to have them carried out should always be undertaken with this remote possi-

Table 33
Routine Vaccinations, Their Possible Side Effects,
and Individuals for Whom Contraindicated

Vaccination	Possible side effects	Contraindicated for
Whooping cough (pertussis)	Encephalitis, death; exacerbate asthma	Children with asthma
Diphtheria	Local irritation	People with diphtheria-toxoid allergy
Tetanus	Local irritation	People with tetanus allergy
Polio	*Very* rarely polio occurs	
Measles	Encephalitis	Severe eczema; people with reduced immunity; people allergic to eggs
German measles	Encephalitis, birth defects	Severe eczema; people with reduced immunity
Smallpox*	Encephalitis, discriminated "smallpox" disease	Everyone, due to risk and disappearance of smallpox

*Not recommended anymore.

bility in mind. These routine vaccinations, their possible side effects, and the individuals for whom they might be contraindicated are outlined in Table 33.

Reactions to Oral or Topical Medications

One of the advantages of medications given by injection is that they must be administered by the provider or surrogate. This maximizes the possibility of delivering a proper dosage and detecting reactions early. (It also, let it be said, runs the risk of causing fainting in some individuals who have a phobic dread of the needle; if this applies to you, let the fact be known.) With medications delivered orally or topically, the controls wither away.

Almost any medication, whether prescription or over-the-counter, can cause a reaction in a susceptible person. Even the most popular, most esteemed, most widely used drugs present risks. Aspirin "...the wonder drug that works wonders..." represents a serious danger to allergy sufferers, especially asthmatics; so does theophylline, a specific asthma medication whose level in the blood must be monitored and adjusted carefully so that it remains both effective and safe. Sleeping pills, cold remedies, and psychotropic drugs (tranquilizers), either alone or in concert with alcohol or other depressants, can trigger dangerous reactions. Some drugs, such as cortisone, are inherently dangerous, causing massive side effects, and ought to be avoided unless medical opinion absolutely dictates their use. With so many drugs on the market, the only way we can guide you is to outline a conservative strategy for the use of oral or topical medications. We suggest:

1. Avoid taking drugs if at all possible. (Many ordinary complaints will respond to nonchemical measures; others, such as the common cold, are not much affected by medications, or the medications themselves carry undesirable side effects.)
2. Before taking any medication, consult the *Physician's Desk Reference* (PDR) for a listing of its

dangers and side effects. (The PDR can be found in your doctor's office, HMO, or the reference section of your local library.) Use the first sections of the book to identify and locate the medications you want to find out more about.

3. Carefully read the directions for use of the medication and follow them exactly. Do not overdose. If a course of treatment is prescribed, carry it through to completion even though your symptoms get better or go away before the prescription runs out.

4. If you develop a reaction to the drug, call your doctor at once.

5. Never use medications for conditions other than the ones for which they were prescribed.

6. Never use anyone else's medication for any condition. (When the need for a prescription is over, it is a good idea to dispose of the leftover pills, or whatever, appropriately so that you won't succumb to the temptation to use them for other ailments for which they were not intended or to pass them on to someone else.)

7. Many widely advertised, over-the-counter medications—cold remedies, nasal sprays, sleep aids, skin care preparations, etc.—combine ineffectiveness and high cost with addictive properties and the possibility of side effects. To paraphrase an old saw, the person who medicates himself has a fool for a patient. And, seeing a drug advertised on TV is, in itself, a good enough reason for avoiding it. (When the advertised drug is useful, its exact generic equivalent can be found a few feet down the pharmacist's shelves at a fraction of the advertised product's cost.)

8. The question "Are you allergic to any drugs or medications?" is routinely asked whenever a treatment is prescribed or administered. There are a couple of problems implicit in the query. First, most people don't really know whether they are sensitive to or have unknowingly been sensitized to a drug through prior use and reply "No" instead of the more accurate "Don't know." Second, the information is called for perfunctorily and in some instances goes unnoticed or unheeded. There are cases on record in which individuals who actually reported adverse reactions to a particular drug were, in fact, given that drug with serious consequences. If you know that a drug causes a reaction in you, state that fact firmly and be sure beforehand that whatever is prescribed for your condition is not a member of the offending drug's family. If the reaction is potentially dangerous, get and wear a Medic-Alert bracelet or necklace. *See* Appendix N for how to get this useful adjunct to medical care.

Reciting all of these "dos and don'ts" may seem to be unnecessary and tiresome, but the facts are that many people are made ill by medicines and taking an inappropriate medicine, or one that provokes a reaction, can carry tragic consequences.

A Note on Anaphylaxis

Anaphylaxis—a serious, frightening, and sometimes fatal shock reaction—can be triggered by a number of antigens. The response occurs with amazing swiftness—sometimes in a few seconds—and is marked by some or all of the following symptoms:

- Wheezing and respiratory compromise
- Swelling or edema of mucous tissue in the mouth and throat
- Sudden and sharp drop in blood pressure
- Massive outbreak of hives
- Feelings of faintness, even loss of consciousness
- Nausea and vomiting
- Behavioral symptoms including confusion, intense anxiety, or vague, unfocused feelings of dread.

Anaphylaxis is popularly identified with bee stings, but injections—allergy shots, novocaine, penicillin, other medications—and many foods can provoke the shock reaction.

Anaphylaxis is acutely dangerous and demands an immediate response. This usually entails injecting epinephrine—which reverses the drop in blood pressure—and giving antihistamines to nullify the histamine release, which is the core of the problem. If you have a history of a shock reaction you should carry and know how to use an ANA-Kit or an Epi-Pen; these can be purchased with a prescription from your doctor. You should also wear Medic-Alert identification to warn medical personnel of the existence of your condition and to point to appropriate steps to take to help you in the event of an emergency. The address of the MedicAlert Foundation is given in Appendix N.

Dangers in the Health Care Setting

Gottlieb is in the hospital for a hernia repair. The operation is routine and uneventful, but when he is returned to his room, Gottlieb complains about a painful burning from the back of his head to his buns. The nurse helps him to roll over and discovers that his whole back is severely inflamed. She reports this to the doctor, who prescribes an ointment that offers some relief. The symptoms gradually fade away in a couple of days, and the doctor, mystified at first, checks and runs some tests on Gottlieb and finds that he is extremely sensitive to the agent used to clean the operating table.

Medical and dental offices, hospitals, and clinics bulge with chemicals, agents, and devices ancillary to treatment that are capable of triggering a wide range of problems. In most instances the patients are shielded from inadvertent contact with these substances, but occasionally they do cause problems. And there are some adjuncts to treatment that do carry risk.

Joe Bob's employer adopts a new dental plan for his employees. Joe Bob goes to the new dentist for a checkup and cleaning, and the dentist, using a probe, locates a superficial gum-line cavity that has lost its filling. (Joe Bob brushes and flosses religiously and has had no problems other than broken fillings for over 20 years.) The dentist then tells Joe Bob that he needs to do a series of X-rays. Joe Bob says that he had such a series by the previous provider 2 years back, that he doesn't think he needs the pictures, that the risk is unacceptable to him, and that he will supply the old films. The dentist says he must have a new set. Joe Bob refuses to allow himself to be put through a new series of six X-rays, saying that he can see no reason from them apart from the fact that they will enable the dentist to charge the insurance company for them. The dentist tells Joe Bob that he does not want Joe Bob for a patient. Joe Bob tells the dentist that he does not want him for a dentist. They part.

Listing all the different substances or agents that can turn up in health care settings and the problems they can cause is beyond the scope of this book. We suggest that you guard against this risk by being completely briefed on the procedures you will undergo, that you have any associated risks explained to you in full and so that you can understand them, and that there are emergency countermeasures in place and ready for deployment. Also, be certain that your care provider knows any details of your health history that might bear on the mode of treatment selected. Wherever possible, opt for the most conservative procedures available that are consistent with your condition.

Points to Remember

The doctor's office, the clinic, and the hospital are particularly dangerous places for individuals with irritant sensitivities or allergies. If you are such a person, be sure that your health care provider knows that. If you need treatment, make an informed choice of the alternative that carries the fewest risks for you. When there are no options, and risk in some degree is present, satisfy yourself that there are emergency procedures in place and instantly accessible to trained personnel. Temper the high degree of trust that you invest in health care providers with the knowledge that mistakes or misjudgments occur, and that they can be largely avoided if you are aware of exactly what is to be done and review each step in the treatment procedure with the individual or individuals providing the service. If there is an inability or unwillingness to display this sort of candor, think about finding another source of help for your health care.

CHAPTER 15

Travel, School, and on the Road

"Let's get away from it all," the once popular song pleads. But one thing you can't flee is the presence of allergens or irritants whose magic spell, like love's, is everywhere.

Any irritant that bothers you at home can also turn up when you're out and about—and the bad news is that there may be other irritants out there you don't normally run into at home that can spring up to give you trouble.

You already know what to do about problems that crop up at home or on the job. Here are some points it may pay to be alert to as you travel (near or far), attend school, or just go about your errands.

Travel

Travel to distant places poses a couple of risks to the irritant- or allergy-prone individual. The first risk has to do with the means of travel itself.

Air travel may expose you to tobacco smoke and irritant airborne chemicals. Airports themselves will likely have a heavy concentration of particulate matter in the air; the fumes from incompletely burned jet

fuel are an unavoidable part of air travel. If you react
to tobacco smoke, fly a carrier that bans smoking.
Domestic flights of 6 hours or less in the United States
do not allow smoking, but international flights on most
carriers still allow cigarets in the rear sections of all
cabin partitions. At some foreign ports of entry, the
cabins (and passengers) may be sprayed with insecticides before passengers are allowed to debark. Inquire
in advance about this possibility and carry a particu-
late-arresting mask in your cabin luggage if you're
going to get zapped with bug spray.

Air travel will also expose you to airline cuisine,
which is probably not as disastrous as some critics
charge, although it is laced with fat, preservatives,
food colors, and other accoutrements of fast-food fare.
Unless you plan ahead, what you get is the standard
offering for the day. However, by calling 48 or more
hours in advance of departure, you can order any of a
large variety of special diets—milk-free, low salt, low-
fat, kosher, vegetarian, Hindu, and seafood, among
others—depending on the carrier and the destination.
And, if you have any qualms about the food you are
served, don't eat it.

Travel by surface (rail, bus, or automobile) can
expose you to emissions and pollens, as well as the
risks inherent in fast-food cuisine. To minimize these
dangers, try to travel at times when the plants that
affect you are not pollenating. If traveling by private
automobile, keep the windows closed and use the air
conditioner (if you have one) to screen out particulate
matter. Do not allow others to smoke in the car; smoking has been outlawed by Amtrak and Greyhound, the
principal surface common carriers.

Insofar as food sensitivities or allergies are concerned, follow the precautions about dining out that are spelled out in Chapters 6 and 10.

Arthur, 11, has chronic asthma that is well-controlled, providing he takes his medication and uses his Pulmo-Aide. His asthma has been so stable over a period of time that his family decides that a trip to England holds no risks. They pack all of Arthur's medication including his Pulmo-Aide and hand carry everything on the airplane. What they simply overlook is that their model of Pulmo-Aide will not work on English voltage, and when Arthur has an episode shortly after they arrive, they have a hard time treating him. If they had carried along the appropriate electrical transformer (or a battery pack model of the device), Arthur would have been completely protected.

Once reached, the destination, whether intermediate or final, may offer risks that, if unanticipated, can be troublesome. Especially prevalent are airborne allergens or irritants, such as pollens, animal danders, molds, and dust.

We have already recommended that, if you are sensitive to pollens, you limit your travel to times of the year or to locations where your particular nemesis is not to be found.

A few individual motels and hotels are taking a more aggressive interest in the health and well-being of their guests and maintain tobacco or pet-free rooms. Look for such facilities by booking your stay through one of the larger chains (Best Western; Holiday Inn; Sheraton, etc). However, most hostelries do not provide such facilities, and a fair share of them are indifferently cleaned, so that they are quite likely to support thriving colonies of mold and mites. The best you can do here is to ask to inspect the room before renting, to inquire about policies regarding pets, to find out about the use of fabric softeners (if you react to them as some do) in their laundering, and to see whether they employ scented air fresheners or other possible sources of trouble in the cleaning process. If you don't like what you hear, see, or smell, decline to rent. (Watch out for shag carpeting, dust along moldings or under pieces of furniture, musty fabric curtains or wall hangings, and mold in bathrooms, especially in shower stalls and underneath or around fixtures.) Kits to test for the quantity of dust and to detect the presence of animal dander are available, but have not been well-studied yet. As of this time, we do not routinely recommend their use.

There are a few simple precautions you can take to remove much of the travail from travel:

- Take your medications with you. Keep them on your person or in a place that is readily and immediately accessible.
- Be alert to the possibility of environmental threats en route to, at, and returning from your destination and make plans, in advance, to circumvent them.
- Wear Medic-Alert identification if this is necessary in your case.
- Insist that your carrier maintain conditions that will not put you at risk.
- Complain where necessary, not only to the company, but to its regulatory agencies.

Special Precautions for Children

One trend of the times is for children to "sleep over"—to stay at a friend's house overnight. If your child is allergic or susceptible to irritants, you should take all the necessary steps beforehand to see that he or she is not going to be exposed to the trigger or, if exposure does occur, the hosts know what counter-measures to take. In particular be alert to the possibility of the presence of animal dander. The dander, even from outdoor-dwelling pets can be transported into the house in a variety of ways and may pose a significant threat to a severely sensitive youngster. In addition teach your child—even a young child, 4–5 years old—the steps to take in the event something happens away from home. The world is full of pitfalls and kids have a way of falling into them.

Chrissy recently went to the RAD, a popular and lively weekend teen center and disco in a small town in Georgia. The hall was illuminated with bright flashing lights and, at one point during the evening, to spice up the glitzy atmosphere a pressurized can of instant fog was released on the dance floor. Although the label clearly stated that this material should not be inhaled by anyone with asthma, Chrissy, who was dancing up a storm at the time the canister went off, got a lungful of the stuff. Almost immediately she went into a severe attack that her medication would not ease. Knowing she was in trouble, she was able to tell the manager of her plight. The manager called an ambulance immediately and Chrissy went to the emergency room, where her symptoms were treated.

School

Anything that can provoke a sensitivity or allergic reaction at home can be found at school—plus a few complications. In addition to potential problems with school food or exposure to harsh soaps, molds, dust, and ill-maintained heating or air conditioning systems, schools offer some special hazards.

Contact dermatitis frequently results from materials encountered in art or shop classes—paints and pigments, resins, clays, solders, fluxes, glues, mastics, chromate, etc. (Strategies to follow in avoiding or managing the symptoms most of these materials cause are spelled out in Chapter 12.)

Laboratory chemicals and gases can be potent triggers of respiratory or cutaneous distress. Some of the more ubiquitous offenders are, among the gases, hydrogen sulfide and sulfur dioxide. Chemicals often implicated in skin disorders include benzene and carbon tetrachloride. In large measure problems originating with these substances can be managed through adequate venting supplemented by use of appropriate safety equipment—masks to filter out particulate material, protective gear including safety glasses, gloves, and so on. One complication crops up when students, not wishing to make themselves conspicuous in the eyes of their peers, choose not to observe precautions they ought to be following. The teacher should be made aware of any problems your child has; the child should be taught by you to put his or her health and safety ahead of appearances.

Exercise-induced asthma is a fairly common phenomenon. Hard, sustained periods of physical exer-

tion, especially under dry or cold conditions, can provoke the characteristic cough and wheeze of asthma.
In our experience, this form of asthma (indeed, all
forms of asthma) is not well-understood by physical
education teachers, who seem prone to believe that
the symptoms are either psychologically rooted or put
on by malingerers.

> Ellen's gym teacher told her that she must run
> laps with the other students, even though a let-
> ter from Ellen's parents and a doctor's statement
> said she could not do this sort of exercise. The
> teacher told Ellen that if she got into the running
> the wheezing would go away. The teacher had that
> one wrong and the school had to pick up the tab
> for the emergency room visit.

Errant school policies often make life difficult for
allergic or hypersensitive youngsters. In many institu-
tions school regulations outlaw the carrying or use of
medications, particularly inhalers used to deliver beta
agonists. As a parent it is your responsibility to bring
your child's problem to the notice of school officials and
to work out, in advance, a procedure wherein a prompt
and effective response can be made in the event of
need. An appropriate procedure may entail providing
a physician's statement attesting to the problem and
specifying effective countermeasures, giving parental
permission for treatment, and working out a treatment strategy with school personnel—administrators,
teachers, counselors, and health personnel.

Exposure to or use of illicit substances, especially
alcohol, drugs, and tobacco, can also provoke reactions
in susceptible students and drugs are an ugly fact of
life in most school settings. Here, responsibility for

avoiding these triggers rests equally with the family and the child. In particular the child needs to be taught not only to steer clear of the substance, whatever it is, but should be helped to develop ways of resisting peer pressure. Talking openly about the dangers attendant to drug use is important; so is teaching strategies for dealing with the child's contemporaries and reinforcing successful efforts at resisting experimentation with or use of these substances. Parental behavior that provides an affirmative model for children to follow is also desirable.

Allergies and School Performance

"Allergies," especially those said to arise from vague or ill-defined causes that result in diffuse symptoms like chronic fatigue, headaches, anxiety, and so forth, are often blamed for poor school performance. We are regularly asked to examine students with failing school records to determine whether an allergy is responsible for their low grades.

Although it is true that allergies (by causing frequent absences from school, or torpor or inattentiveness resulting from the side effects of medications like antihistamines) can sometimes be associated with poor school performance, we almost never find that previously undiagnosed allergies, in and of themselves, account for poor grades. In fact, visual or auditory problems are much more likely to be at the root of underachievement. Moreover, so far as we know, allergies play no role whatsoever in behavioral difficulties in school—attention deficits, hyper- or hypoactivity in the classroom, discipline problems, and the like.

If your child *is* allergic and chronically symptomatic and takes certain medications, his or her grades *may* suffer as a result. But looking to allergies as a cause of poor grades in a child who has been historically free of symptoms is grasping at straws. "Allergy" is a catchword; Charlie Brown (and too many real-life children) declare that they are allergic to math, for instance. More accurately, they may not be apt in math, but the likelihood is that they (and, all too often, their parents) have a learned and reinforced negative attitude toward the subject. That is not an allergy—it is a disorder or a disability that calls for other than allergic countermeasures.

Allergies and Getting the Most Out of Life

From what we have said in this chapter, so far, it would be easy to conclude that allergies or irritant sensitivities put a damper on everything. Though these vulnerabilities can cause problems and force limitation of some activities in some people, it will pay you to remember:

* Careful observation of avoidance strategies almost certainly will keep you out of serious trouble.
* Continual refinement and improvement in medications is constantly enlarging opportunities for enjoyable participation in most aspects of a full life.
* Although some activities may be denied to you, there are substitutes you can engage in that are safe, enjoyable, and rewarding. You can find a way around your problem; there is no need to be enslaved by it.

Not so long ago children with allergies—especially asthmatics—were routinely kept from attending summer camp. Now, with advances in treatment, plus a better understanding of the nature of asthmatic disease, asthmatics can now participate in and enjoy the camp experience. And, for children who have severe asthmatic or other respiratory problems, the American Lung Association now offers sponsored camps designed especially for those youngsters in most regions of the country. The children thrive in those settings; they develop confidence in their ability to manage their symptoms, they learn from other children how to deal with their condition and, meanwhile, their parents get some needed respite from the daily burden of care. Your asthmatic or allergy-prone child may not wind up as one, but it is surprising and immensely encouraging to note how many world-class athletes in a variety of sports—and stars in other fields of endeavor—are asthmatic or troubled with other atopic diseases.

Points to Remember

You *can* take your allergies or hypersensitivities with you. With the right kind of forethought and planning, you can anticipate and avoid the problems that may crop up away from home—at school, while visiting, or while traveling. The points to remember are these:

1. *Be prepared.* Carry your medications and have them on your person or close at hand so that they can be put into play as soon as they are needed. Formulate emergency tactics in advance of the moment of need.

2. Be alert. Insofar as possible determine the risks you are likely to encounter, institute appropriate avoidance tactics, and stick to them unswervingly.

3. Be prudent. Most likely you can safely do what other folks do when they are away from home, but try not to trust to luck or push the limits.Don't take chances or play games with your condition.

4. Be fair. Try not to blame allergies for personal shortcomings or use them as an excuse for inactivity or poor performance. The fault may well lie elsewhere.

CHAPTER 16

Sick Building Syndromes

Some environments have long been known to be unhealthy for the people who have to spend time in them. Mines, foundries, chemical plants, and even farms are often associated with a high incidence of respiratory or cutaneous ailments. The symptoms, in these milieus, result directly from exposure to substances that are an integral part of the activities or processes being conducted in the environment.

In the last 15 years or so there have been increasing numbers of reports of epidemic outbreaks of symptoms associated with the properties of buildings themselves. This phenomenon has been variously called tight building syndrome, sick building syndrome, building sickness, or ill building. Obviously, the building itself is not "sick"; the people who live or (more likely) work in it are the ones who display the symptoms. However, features of the building itself or its occupants may be the triggers.

The incidence of building-related symptoms is tied to the change in the nature and composition of the work force, the construction of energy-efficient buildings, and drastic reductions in the minimum recommended air exchange rate.

With the energy crisis of the 1970s (and the growing emphasis on the "bottom line" idolized by Harvard

237

MBAs), energy efficiency became a dominant theme in commercial building design and construction. The resulting structures are predominantly commercial or governmental office buildings, but universities, public schools, and even hospitals also went up for which a major design goal was to achieve a uniform, controlled indoor climate that would require minimal cost for its operation and upkeep. In practical terms this meant building a tight, well-insulated structure with a mechanically/electronically controlled climate requiring the smallest possible indoor ventilation rate.[1] At the same time the nature and composition of the work force was changing—proportionately and absolutely many more clerical, service, white-collar workers, more women—so that a higher percentage of the work force could be found in these burgeoning, sealed, climate-controlled, often windowless cubes. The result was an eruption of reports of epidemic illness among people who worked in these monuments to technology and maximized profit.

The air supply is, in a sense, invariant; indeed, some find a measure of satisfaction in pointing out that any lungful of air might include a molecule once breathed by Jesus Christ, Genghis Khan, Catherine the Great, or Sweeney Todd.

In a tight building the air supply is largely recycled, and thus much more closed than in times gone

---

[1]The minimum indoor ventilation rate recommended by the American Society of Heating, Refrigerating, and Air Conditioning Engineers has seen a sixfold drop in the past 80 years. Their original turn-of-the-century standard of a minimum rate of 30 ft^3/min was reduced, finally, to the current 5 ft^3/min in 1973.

by. Moreover, the construction of the building itself may directly compromise the quality of the air in it. Air pollution can arise from malfunctioning or ill-maintained air conditioning equipment, emissions from the building materials, the furnishings, or the office machines, as well as from the effluvia of human metabolism and from ambient outdoor pollutants. Thus, in the tight building, much of what is in the air is continually recirculated, just as is the often foul air in passenger jets. In fact, working in a tight building might sometimes seem like spending eight hours a day in a passenger jet without the noise and flight attendants. Though maintained at a reasonable temperature, the air in these structures is neither fresh, clean, nor uncontaminated.

The number of buildings investigated by public health officials in connection with the outbreak of mass symptomatology among workers has risen sharply in the last decade and a half. Three-quarters of those investigations were of large, recently constructed, airtight, energy-efficient office buildings.

Symptoms and Causes of Building-Related Illness

Building-related illness most often is expressed in the respiratory system. Some of the respiratory symptoms may be allergic—asthma or hay fever in particular; others result from infection. Skin irritation or irritation of mucous membranes, particularly those of the eyes, nose, and throat, occur and may be accompanied by headache, lethargy, and vague feelings of malaise, fatigue, dizziness, or drowsiness.

Building-Related Respiratory Allergies

Energy-efficient buildings contribute to the production of asthma or hay fever symptoms in a number of important ways. Maintaining a high level of relative humidity provides an ideal climate for the propagation of dust mites and mold, which are important triggers for these diseases. Dust mites, as we point out in Chapter 12, are important airborne triggers of respiratory allergies. These creatures can be controlled by holding the relative humidity below 50%; however, the individual's perceived level of comfort depends on both temperature and humidity. (At a given thermometer reading it will seem warmer if the humidity is kept high.) Therefore, in an energy-efficient structure the humidity is kept elevated (during the cool seasons) to realize fuel cost savings. The result is a climate ideal for the propagation of mites.

The same high level of humidity also fosters growth of the molds and fungi that can cause asthma and rhinitis. Quite often these triggers flourish inside humidifying equipment that not only moistens the air, but distributes it impartially throughout the structure, often producing cases of "humidifier asthma." Air conditioning and humidifying equipment require regular maintenance and frequent and scrupulous cleaning if they are to be kept from broadcasting allergic triggers.

Other less important sources of mold include office plants. New-age office buildings seem to have replaced honest, old-fashioned file cabinets and calendar decor with extravagant displays of greenery that can be the dank source of a myriad of spores. Double-paned fixed windows promote condensation on the frames, and these persistent moist spots frequently harbor thriving patches of mildew or mold. Leaks in the roof or plumbing, or liquid spills on "industrial" carpeting (a cheap to install and maintain, but ultimately ugly alternative to a real floor) also provide congenial spots for the growth of molds.

Energy-efficient structures have also been implicated in the development of hypersensitivity pneumonitis and humidifier fever. These relatively uncommon conditions result from an immune system-mediated inflammation of the lower airways. A substantial list of fungi, bacteria, and protozoa have been identified as the triggers for these essentially respiratory allergies. The microorganisms that trigger the symptoms multiply in a microbial slime that builds up in air conditioning or humidifying systems and are dispersed throughout the building, affecting susceptible persons.

With hypersensitivity pneumonitis, the symptoms can vary widely, depending on the level of vulnerability of the individual and the degree of exposure to the antigen. They may include shortness of breath, a dry cough, flu-like symptoms, including fever and headache, acute bouts of inflammation of the lung or, over a period of time, buildup of fibrous tissue in the lungs.

Humidifier fever typically results in flu-like symptoms, such as fever, chills, headache, chest tightness, and breathing difficulty, appearing on the evening of the first day following return to work after an absence. Symptoms usually subside within 12 hours and do not return until the next work day following later days off.

The construction materials and furnishings of a new building can represent an additional source of trouble. Asthma or other respiratory complaints do result from emissions from insulation, plywood or particle board, plastics, mastics, adhesives, synthetic fibers, and a host of other building materials (*see* Chapters 11 and 12). Dry detergent residue used to shampoo carpets has been implicated in outbreaks of respiratory trouble, and there is a mounting body of evidence that tight buildings promote photochemical reactions that produce the precursors of aldehyde, formaldehyde, hydrocarbon vapors, and the like. That means that you can have smog whether you're crawling down the freeway or jockeying your desk.

Beyond mites, molds, and fungi, tobacco smoke (which, in closed environments where smoking is permitted, will be recirculated democratically so that you and all your fellow-workers share the boss' stogie) represents a hazard to allergy-prone individuals, as do unusual smells. Pungent vapors from chemicals, perfumes, colognes, and after-shave lotions borne by colleagues persist stubbornly in these "controlled" environments and can sensitize you to the point where allergic symptoms appear.

Your allergic symptoms likely result from conditions in the place where you work if they appear only during (or after) work, disappear on vacations and days off, and (excepting humidifier fever) intensify during the work week. If these features characterize your symptoms, follow the steps outlined in Chapters 4 and 15 to identify and eliminate the triggers.

Respiratory Infections

The modern, tight office building also provides a congenial breeding ground for organisms that cause respiratory infections. Outbreaks of colds or flu that hit almost an entire office or school classroom population seem to be more prevalent than was true in earlier times. It seems quite plausible to attribute this newfound catholicity of certain illnesses to closed systems that recycle germ-laden air.

In addition, several infectious syndromes are specifically tied to poor circulation, and faulty or poorly maintained air conditioning equipment. The diseases are Legionnaires' disease, Pontiac fever, and Q fever. All of these diseases are triggered by bacteria primarily contaminating cooling equipment, although hot water pipes, shower heads, humidifiers, condensers, ice machines, and respiratory therapy equipment may harbor the organisms as well.

Legionnaires' disease and Pontiac fever can be caused by any one of a number of different bacilli. The incidence of these diseases is probably grossly underreported; estimates are that 70,000 cases and 1000 fatalities are chargeable each year to the pneumonic form of Legionnaires' disease alone. Pontiac fever, the nonpneumonic form, is less virulent, but much more contagious, than Legionnaires' disease; the attack rate runs 95% with a 3-day incubation period.

Q-fever has also been associated with closed buildings. Rickettsia-caused, it produces flu-like symptoms. The reservoirs for the causal organism are infected laboratory animals colonies maintained at university or research laboratory complexes.

Dermatitis

Building-related dermatitis can usually be suspected if several employees in an office develop skin rashes and intense itching in exposed parts of the body. People who wear contact lenses will also experience intense eye discomfort with copious tearing. Its cause is almost always traceable to fiberglass insulation.

When damaged by hard use, repair work, or water, the fiberglass material used to insulate ventilation ducts breaks down and minute particles are released—through the climate control system—to fall equally on the susceptible and the unsusceptible alike. (Work-related dermatitis that results from handling materials on the job was covered in Chapter 13.) Building-related dermatitis can usually be controlled by installing HEPA screens over vents and by replacing damaged insulation.

Irritation of Mucous Membranes

The most commonly reported symptoms attributed to tight buildings—and the ones most difficult to trace to a specific cause—are those involving annoyance or irritation of the mucous membranes. The symptoms that have been associated with energy-efficient buildings at one time or another are listed in Table 34.

Firmly establishing any of these symptoms as building-linked presents a problem since they have so many other possible causes. In addition, self reports of illness are influenced by differences in individuals' perceptions of wellness, the nature of the work environment, and the job activities or duties themselves. People performing dull, repetitive tasks more often complain of symptoms like the ones tabled below than do workers carrying out varied, interesting tasks.

Table 34
Symptoms Associated with Mucous Membrane
Irritation and Tight Buildings

Sneezing	Eye irritation, watering
Chest tightness	Nasal congestion, sinus stuffiness
Nausea	Fatigue
Dry throat	Dizziness
Drowsiness	Dry, nonproductive cough
Headache	Problem wearing contact lenses

If the place of work is involved, the symptoms will usually be shortlived, will intensify during the work day, will improve rapidly after the employee leaves the building, and will variously affect a number of workers in the same physical area of the building.

Mass Psychogenic Illness

Headmasters and headmistresses at schools throughout East and Central Africa dread the outbreak of the "laughing sickness." Every year a few schools will have to shut down completely because the pupils will be overcome by persistent, uncontrollable fits of laughing. The condition becomes epidemic to the point where carrying out normal school activities is impossible and the children must be sent home for a time. These outbreaks have no apparent cause.

Epidemic outbreaks of illness not traceable to any chemical or microbial cause are frequently associated with (and blamed on) tight buildings. Symptoms can take a wide variety of forms, including headaches, dizziness, dry throat, sore eyes, metallic taste, disorientation, nausea, fatigue, or even fainting or convulsions.

Application of the "psychogenic" label to these kinds of outbreaks should be done only after exhaustive analysis, not only of the physical properties of the workplace itself, but of the nature and conditions of work. When the tasks are dull, confining, and repetitive, carried out under poor physical conditions, under strict authoritarian pressure, or are otherwise stressful, these conditions themselves may provoke reports of illness. Yet, most cases of alleged tight building syndrome that are investigated do not turn up a specific cause or causes for the outbreak of illness. This may be because there is no physical cause, the physical cause (whatever it is) is not detectable given the existing state of our knowledge, or it exists in the psychological environment of the employees. Whatever the cause, however, the symptoms experienced by the employee are real and affect performance on the job.

Points to Remember

Well over 300 instances of building-associated illness have been investigated by the United States Public Health Service and by Health and Welfare Canada in the past decade. Slightly more than half of these investigations found the buildings to be inadequately ventilated, although this condition itself could not account for the symptoms displayed by the workers. The melancholy fact is that about four-fifths of the air in a modern, tight building is recycled or recirculated. Bringing in and heating (or cooling) fresh outdoor air represents a substantial cost. Since the air is recycled, it offers an excellent opportunity for contamination to build up, especially if the system is shut down overnight or on weekends.

Other important causes of building-associated sickness were found to be the circulation of outside contaminants and contaminants built or brought into the structure itself (building materials and furnishings). No identifiable problem turned up in a bit over ten percent of the buildings studied.

PART 6

HELP SOURCES AND RESOURCES

CHAPTER 17

Private and Public
Sources of Help

*Allergists, Dermatologists, Pulmonary Specialists,
Neurologists, Industrial Health Consultants,
and HESIS, OSHA, Worker's Compensation,
Insurance Carriers, Employer Health and Safety
Officer, and so on*

We cannot repeat often enough that the trick to managing allergic or irritant-sensitive reactions is to identify whatever it is that triggers your symptoms and then to avoid it religiously. Fortunately, most people either have a very good idea of the source of their difficulties, or can gain one by carefully following the procedures we spell out in Chapter 4. If you haven't been able to nail down the source of your difficulties, one reason may be that you are uniquely susceptible to what is ordinarily an innocuous and innocent-appearing agent.

> Sandi's mild asthma suddenly intensified and became very persistent despite aggressive treatment with drugs and inhalants. Her allergist was finally able to establish that the wintergreen flavoring in the tartar-control toothpaste to which she had recently switched was responsible for her wheezing. As soon as she went back to her origi-

251

nal dentifrice, her symptoms improved dramatically. It turns out that she didn't even have to worry about tartar buildup. The ingredients in the two products (by the same manufacturer) are exactly the same, except for the artificial flavorings employed.

Other hard-to-unearth causes may be associated with intermittent exposure to the agent, the need to have a significant level of exposure for the symptoms to show, and infections or disease. When you don't know and can't seem to unearth whatever it is that is causing your symptoms, you are at a point where you need outside help. Here are the people and places you can turn to.

Your Family Doctor

The first place to look for help is your family physician. To get the most benefit from this resource, prepare carefully for the appointment by gathering as much information as you can about your symptoms—what form they take, when, where, and under what circumstances they appear, how long they last, what seems to intensify them or make them worse. It will also help if you can supply information on your activities and daily routines before the symptoms showed. (The schedules in Chapter 4, if kept carefully, will be useful, especially if they are maintained faithfully, rather than for just a few days or intermittently.)

The physician should supplement the information you provide with a complete physical examination and an exhaustive health history. If these activities are carried out perfunctorily or not done at all, that may be a signal to look for another doctor.

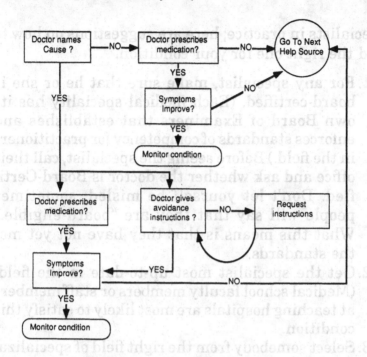

Fig. 7. Front-line medical procedures in the diagnosis and treatment of allergen or irritant-caused disease.

With the examination and history completed, the doctor (and you) will likely follow a chain or sequence of steps and arrive at the conclusions sketched in Figure 7.

Your family doctor may or may not be able to help you. If he or she does, fine; if not, move on to the next help source—usually a medical specialist.

Consulting a Specialist

To line up a specialist, the best place to start is with your own family doctor. Simply tell your physician that you would like a second opinion or referral. There are literally scores of different kinds of medical specialists in practice; here are suggestions on how to find the right one for your condition.

1. For any specialist, make sure that he or she is board-certified. (Each medical speciality has its own Board of Examiners that establishes and enforces standards of competency for practitioners in the field.) Before seeing the specialist, call their office and ask whether the doctor is Board-Certified. Don't let yourself be misled; sometimes people will say that they are "board-eligible." What this means is that they have not yet met the standards.

2. Get the specialist most up-to-date in the field. (Medical school faculty members or staff members at teaching hospitals are most likely to satisfy this condition.

3. Select somebody from the right field of specialization. The person you will see depends on the symptoms you have been suffering. Here is what we suggest:

Condition	Appropriate specialist
Allergic diseases (asthma, hay fever, eczema)	Allergist
Contact dermatitis	Dermatologist/allergist
Gastric problems	Gastroenterologist
Hives	Dermatologist/allergist
Severe respiratory problems	Pulmonologist/allergist
Joint pains	Rheumatologist

At this stage, be careful that you are not referred to someone whose specialty does not address problems apparently brought on by allergens or irritants; internists, ENT doctors, psychiatrists, and so on are unlikely to be of much help to you.

Table 35
Routine Tests for Causes of Allergen or Irritant-Related Symptoms

Symptoms	Tests	Comment
Asthma	Skin,[1] RAST[3]	May exacerbate symptoms
Hay fever	Skin, RAST	Unreliable when symptoms present
Eczema	Elimination diet, RAST	Patch and skin tests risky under some conditions
Gastric	Elimination diet, skin, RAST, oral food challenge	Challenge test must be carefully supervised
Dermatitis	Patch,[2] challenge	Should be done only when you are symptom-free
Hives	Elimination diet	Skin tests are rarely indicated

[1]Skin tests (scratch, prick, intradermal) are given to detect sensitivity to airborne or food allergies.

[2]Patch tests are used to detect sensitivity to materials touched or handled.

[3]RAST (or FAST) tests are in vitro blood tests measuring presence of IgE antibodies. They indicate the likelihood that your symptoms are or are not allergic, but they do not pinpoint the trigger.

4. Take along all the information you can assemble about your condition. In addition to the material you put together for your own physician, check your family background for relatives (parents; aunts and uncles; your own children) who have had a history of allergic or hypersensitive disorders.

When you begin with the specialist, after the usual preliminaries (physical examination, medical history, history of current symptoms) and depending on your condition, you may be subjected to a series of tests or regimens. The ones you may encounter are spelled out in Table 35.

Your specialist—just as you and your family physician did—will try to bring you to the point at which the cause of your symptoms is clearly identified, you know what to do to avoid further exposure, and you can treat yourself appropriately if symptoms recur. The chances are good that a complete and careful review of your case by a specialist will let you know the trigger for your symptoms, how to avoid it, and can treat them competently should they recur. And note well that your insurance carrier or HMO should bear the brunt, if not all, of the costs involved in this sometimes lengthy and costly search for your allergen or irritant. The cost of protective devices, if they are prescribed by a physician, should also be met, at least in part. Unhappily, Medicare, the major health care source for seniors, is considerably less generous about the extent of its support for medical and related services. This is particularly unfortunate because, given the way in which irritant-sensitive or allergic reactions develop, they are prone to be more prevalent and more severe in older persons. The stated policy of Medicare is to purchase durable equipment only when the device is medically necessary and prescribed by a physician (but some environmental control equipment —air cleaners, for instance—are explicitly excluded from coverage.)

There are other resources out there that can also be useful to you. Employers, some state and federal agencies, insurance carriers, trade unions, and private and professional organizations may be in a position to provide you with information and suggestions about locating help and dealing with the cause of your symptoms.

Federal and State Agencies

The governmental agencies most directly concerned with individual health problems of the type discussed in this book are federal and state Occupational Safety and Health Administrations (OSHA). The federal Occupational Safety and Health Act of 1972 established procedures and programs to address safety and health hazards in the workplace. Just how you can utilize this resource depends on the state in which you work; some states maintain their own OSHA programs. In those states, you would make a complaint to the local OSHA office about the workplace condition you suspected was responsible for your illness if you were employed by a private employer or a state or local governmental entity. Complaints by federal employees, and by certain other groups (e.g., maritime workers, residents of Indian reservations, and so on), remain the responsibility of the federal organization.

The law requires that the name of the complainant be held in confidence. The speed with which the complaint is investigated depends on the backlog of cases, but an effort is made to respond with 14 days. Conditions judged to be dangerous are looked into immediately.

In states where there is no state-sponsored OSHA apparatus, the federal statutes and organization assume operating responsibility and should be approached directly. Offices are maintained in most major population centers.

You would complain to state (or federal) OSHA if there was reason for you to believe that your symp-

toms were linked to conditions or materials encountered on the job. To do this, call OSHA under state or
federal government listings in the front part of the
white pages of the telephone directory and tell the
person who answers that you have a health complaint.
Let them advise you from there. A list of OSHA offices is found in Appendix K.

Workers' Compensation Insurance

Most wage-earners are covered by workers' compensation insurance. The coverage may be provided
by public or private carriers; the premiums are paid
by employer and employee contributions. If an illness
is attributable to conditions encountered in the workplace, the insurer will defray medical costs and a percentage of any wages lost owing to absence from the
job caused by work-related illness or injury.

Since the bulk of the insurance cost is borne by
the employer, claims have to be initiated through the
employer. This gives you, the employee, very little
opportunity to initiate action designed to rectify unhealthy or unsafe working conditions. However, compensation insurance carriers do maintain safety de-
partments that conduct investigations of working conditions and can recommend improvements or correc-
tions. A telephone call to that department of the insurance carrier could bring about changes. The most
important thing for you to remember, however, is that
if you are employed, you are (or ought to be) covered
by compensation insurance that should defray medical expenses resulting from job-related illness and pay
some part of your salary when you are off the job for
work-related health reasons.

Trade Unions or Employee Organizations

With reference to work-related illness, unions or employee organizations are obliged to look after the health and welfare of their members. The extent to which they can do this depends importantly on the union and the industry, but our impression is that if an employee believes that his or her allergies or irritant sensitivity is caused by a job-related condition, the approach through the union is tempered by the union–company contract spelling out the conditions of work, and by the union's preoccupation with general issues relating to health and safety. Individual employee complaints are routinely referred to OSHA. Depending on your bargaining agent (if you have one), you may prefer to make the OSHA approach yourself, thus cutting out the middleman, saving some time, and preserving your anonymity.

Employer-Based Health and Safety Programs

Most large, progressive employers provide a number of direct or indirect benefits that may be useful to you in helping you deal with your symptoms.

Company Physicians or Employer-Financed Medical Plans will help defray the costs of treatment of work-related reactions to allergens or irritants. The company doctor, as any other physician, can help you find a cause for and a way of managing your symptoms; your medical insurance will not only pay for treatment but, with the proper medical documentation, will also defray all or most of the costs of any special equipment you may require to keep well—

respirators, air purifiers, particle masks, peak flow meters, spinhalers, gloves, protective clothing, etc. Health and Safety Officers are charged with the responsibility of establishing and maintaining safe work practices. For the most part these officials develop and enforce safety procedures—seeing to it that employees wear or use prescribed safety equipment and that working conditions are kept as nearly hazard-free as possible. However, they are also responsible for looking into other health matters.

> Bernard, the assistant reference librarian in a large metropolitan library developed serious and diffuse symptoms when he returned to work after a lengthy vacation to the Far East. The library was being redecorated and the pattern of Bernard's symptoms at first suggested that he had developed a severe sensitivity reaction to some of the synthetic materials that were being installed—carpets, carpet pads, glues in particular. This suspicion was given weight when, after a period of sick leave and remission of symptoms Bernard returned to work. In the second week following his return he became acutely ill and was taken to the hospital, where his condition worsened and he died. Bernard's colleagues were convinced that he had an acute hypersensitivity reaction to some chemical in the carpeting or its adhesives since there is a lingering pungent odor that still troubles some of them. The city Health and Safety Officer ordered a complete review of the case, which eventually established the cause of death to be an obscure parasitic disease Bernard had apparently contracted while on vacation.

Health and Safety officers are not necessarily experts on health and safety matters—oftentimes they carry this responsibility as an additional duty. But they are the point of contact with both top-level management and OSHA, and they can help to determine whether working conditions are causing your problem and, if they are, to remedy them.

Private Consultants

The past decade has seen the emergence of private consultants, specialists in assessing environmental quality. These individuals or organizations are found in the yellow pages under the Safety Consultants heading. They will, for a fee, evaluate home or work environments and recommend means of eradicating airborne or cutaneous allergens or irritants.

If you need to have your home evaluated (and you would want this done *only* if your own scrupulous investigation had failed to reveal the cause of your problem, *or* your careful attempts at avoidance or control of known triggers had failed), your specialist or HMO may have someone to recommend. Since this is a relatively new field, it will be worth your while to take your time about choosing a consultant; some states require licenses of people who do this type of work. Check to see whether licenses are required in your state, find out whether the firms you are considering hiring are licensed, then go to the licensing bureau and see whether your prospects are licensed and free of prior complaints. Be careful to avoid quacks with little expertise other than a fancy sign on their door.

If you believe your symptoms are job-related, your tactic would be to approach your employer through the appropriate channels (supervisor, shop steward), spelling our your problem, your guess about what might be causing it, and requesting an investigation. The employer is responsible for providing safe working conditions and might respond to your request by (1) ignoring it, countering that adequate health and safety measures were in place, (2) by asking OSHA or Worker's Comp to look into it, or (3) by hiring a private safety consultant. There is an advantage to having a private consultant do the work; it may avoid penalties or insurance rate boosts if there is a risk and a violation. Once the matter has gone forward, however, it is out of your hands.

Other Help Sources

Apart from what we have listed above, there are organizations or agencies that can provide information or direct you to programs that may enable you to manage your symptoms. Here are some of the more accessible and useful ones:

The *American Lung Association* is especially concerned with respiratory problems. They offer a number of programs aimed at helping you to learn more about asthma and to manage your symptoms. They also sponsor stop-smoking clinics. They are in the white pages under American Lung Association.

The *Environmental Protection Agency* (EPA) is more interested in toxins and hazardous materials, but has issued a useful booklet entitled *Removal of Radon from Household Water*. The booklet (which also lists addresses and phone numbers for state radon contacts and EPA regional offices) can be obtained from the United States Environmental Protection Agency,

Washington, DC 20460. The governmental publications section of your local public library should have this document on file.

The *National Asthma Center* in Denver, Colorado has a toll-free number you can call to get information about asthma. The number is 800-222-LUNG.

The *National Asthma Education Program*, 4733 Bethesda Avenue, Suite 530, Bethesda, MD 20814-4820 has a toll-free number, 800-822-ASMA. They will provide information and publications on asthma, hay fever, and dermatitis. They will also be able to direct you to an allergy specialist in your community.

See, also Appendix Q, below, which tells you how and where to find materials or devices you may need to manage your symptoms.

Where Not to Go for Help

Finally, as we have indicated at several points in earlier chapters, there are some helpers that in our view need to be avoided. "Clinical ecologists," specialists in "twentieth-century disease," people who do certain kinds of unproved testing, the practitioners who attribute wide-ranging symptoms to Candida invasions, chiropractors, herbal specialists, homeopaths, hypnotists, and a gallery of practitioners of other esoteric, fad, and almost entirely unproven and ineffectual techniques are all out there waiting to pounce on the unwary or on those made vulnerable by their illness. Avoid them as you would an allergen. Select your helper only after careful deliberation and a review of professional credentials.

APPENDIX A
Common Sites of Mold

Bathroom
1. Leaky fixtures
2. Shower curtains
3. Water pools in window sills
4. Cracks/floor/rugs

Kitchen
1. Leaky fixtures
2. Damp towels
3. Refrigerator drip pans

Other sources in home
1. Virtually anything below ground (i.e., basement)
2. Damp towels, clothing
3. Swamp coolers
4. Vaporizers
5. Garden sheds
6. Compost heaps
7. Garbage disposal
8. Garbage cans

Workplace sites
1. Faulty air conditioners
2. Damp carpets
3. Humidifiers
4. Leaky window sills
5. Damp work areas

APPENDIX B
Pollen Map and Guide for the United States[4]

Map area	Trees[1]	Grasses[2]	Weeds[3]
I CT, ME, MA, NH, NJ, NY, PA, RI, VT	Maple/Box Elder Oak Birch	Timothy Orchard Fescue Redtop	Lamb's Quarter Ragweed, Giant & Short Cocklebur
II DE, DC, MD, NC, VA	Maple/Box Elder Birch Juniper/Cedar	Redtop Vernal grass Bermuda grass Orchard grass Timothy	Pigweed Lamb's Quarter Ragweed, Giant & Short Mexican Firebush
III FL (North) GA, SC	Maple/Box Elder Birch Juniper/Cedar	Redtop Vernal grass Bermuda grass Orchard grass Rye grass	Lamb's Quarter Ragweed, Giant & Short Sagebrush English Plantain
IV FL (South)	Box Elder Oak Juniper/Cedar	Redtop Bermuda grass Salt grass Bahia grass	Pigweed Lamb's Quarter Ragweed, Giant & Short Sagebrush
V IN, KY, OH, TN, WV	Maple/Box Elder Birch Oak Hickory	Redtop Bermuda grass Orchard grass Fescue Rye grass	Waterhemp Pigweed Lamb's Quarter Ragweed, Giant & Short
VI AL, AR, LA, MI	Maple/Box Elder Juniper/ Cedar Oak	Redtop Bermuda grass Orchard grass Rye grass Timothy	Carelessweed/ Pigweed Lamb's Quarter Ragweed, Giant & Short
VII MI, MN, WI	Maple/Box Elder Alder Birch Oak	Redtop Brome Orchard grass Fescue Rye grass	Waterhemp Lamb's Quarter Russian Thistle Ragweed, Giant & Short

(continued...)

Trees-Ash, Birch, Cottonwood,Elder, Elm, Hickory
Grasses- Bermuda grass, Johnson grass, Orchard
grass, Poa spp., Redtop, Timothy
Weeds-Amaranthus spp., Cocklebur, Lamb's Quarter,
Plaintain, Ragweed, Rumex spp.

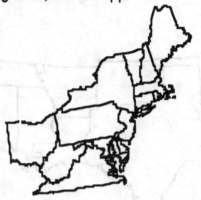

Northeast

Connecticut
Delaware
Maine
Maryland
Massachusetts
New Hampshire
New Jersey
New York
Ohio
Pennsylvania
Rhode Island
Vermont
Virginia
Washington DC
West Virginia

Trees- Ash, Cedar, Cottonwood, Elder, Elm, Oak
Grasses- Bermuda grass, Johnson grass, Orchard
grass, Poa spp., Redtop, Rye, Timothy
Weeds- Amaranthus spp., Cocklebur, Lamb's Quarter
Plaintain, Ragweed, Rumex spp.

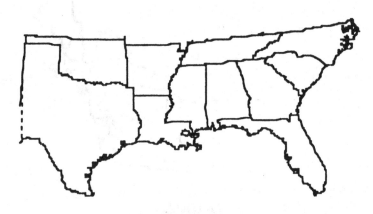

Southeast

Alabama
Arkansas
Florida
Georgia
Louisana
Mississippi
North Carolina
Oklahoma
South Carolina
Tennessee
Texas(Eastern)

Trees-Alder, Birch,Cottonwood,Elder, Elm, Oak
Grasses- Brome, Orchard grass, Redtop, Rye,
    Timothy
Weeds-Amaranthus spp., Lamb's Quarter, Plaintain
    Ragweed, Rumex spp., Sage Brush,
    Saltbush

Northwest

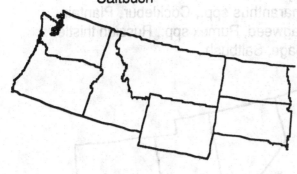

Idaho
Montana
North Dakota
Oregon
South Dakota
Washington
Wyoming

Trees-Ash, Birch,Cottonwood,Elder, Elm, Oak
Grasses- Orchard grass, Redtop, Rye, Timothy
Weeds-Amaranthus spp., Lamb's Quarter, Plaintain
    Ragweed, Rumex spp., Russian Thistle,
    Water Hemp

Midwest

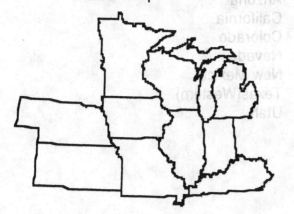

Illinois
Indiana
Iowa
Kansas
Kentucky
Michigan
Minnesota
Missouri
Wisconsin

Trees-Alder, Ash, Birch, Cedar, Cottonwood,
Elder, Elm, Oak, Olive, Sycamore
Grasses- Bermuda grass, Brome, Fescue,
Orchard grass, Poa spp., Redtop,
Rye
Weeds- Amaranthus spp., Cocklebur, Plantain
Ragweed, Rumex spp., Russian thistle
Sage, Saltbush

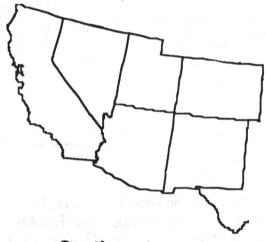

Southwest

Arizona
California
Colorado
Nevada
New Mexico
Texas(Western)
Utah

Pollen Map and Guide
for the United States *(continued)*

Map area	Trees[1]	Grasses[2]	Weeds[3]
VIII IL, IA, MO	Maple/Box Elder Birch Oak Hickory	Redtop Bermuda grass Orchard grass Rye grass Timothy	Pigweed Lamb's Quarter Mexican Firebush Russian Thistle Ragweed, Giant & Short
IX KA, NB, ND, SD	Maple/Box Elder Alder Birch Hazelnut Oak	Quack grass/Waterhemp Wheat grass Redtop Brome Orchard grass Rye grass	Pigweed Lamb's Quarter Mexican Firebush Russian Thistle Ragweed, False, Giant, Short & Western
X OK, TX	Box Elder Juniper/ Cedar Oak Mesquite	Quack grass/ Wheat grass Redtop Bermuda grass Orchard grass	Waterhemp Carelessweed/ Pigweed Saltbush/Scale Lamb's Quarter
XI AZ, CO, ID, MT, NM, UT, WY	Box Elder Alder Birch Juniper/ Cedar Oak	Quack grass/ Wheat grass Redtop Brome Bermuda grass Orchard grass	Waterhemp Pigweed Saltbush/Scale Sugarbeet Lamb's Quarter Mexican Firebush
XII AZ Desert, CA South- eastern Desert	Cypress Juniper/ Cedar Mesquite Ash Olive	Brome Bermuda grass Salt grass Rye grass Canary grass June grass	Carelessweed Iodine Bush Saltbush/Scale Lamb's Quarter Russian Thistle Ragweed, False Slender&Western

(continued...)

Pollen Map and Guide
for the United States (continued)

Map area	Trees[1]	Grasses[2]	Weeds[3]
XIII CA Southern Coastal	Box Elder Cypress Oak Walnut Acacia	Oats Brome Bermuda grass Orchard grass Salt grass	Carelessweed/ Pigweed Saltbush/Scale Lamb's Quarter Russian Thistle Ragweed, False, Slender&Western
XIV CA, Central Valley .	Box Elder Alder Birch Cypress Oak Walnut Olive Ash	Redtop Oats Brome Bermuda grass Rye grass Orchard grass	Pigweed Saltbush/Scale Sugarbeet Lamb's Quarter Russian Thistle Ragweed, False, Slender&Western
XV ID (Southern) NE	Box Elder Alder Birch Juniper/ Cedar Ash	Quack grass/ Wheat grass Redtop Brome Bermuda grass Orchard grass	Pigweed Iodine bush Saltbush/Scale Lamb's Quarter Mexican Firebush Russian Thistle

XVI
OR (Central
& Eastern)
WA (Central
& Eastern)
	Box Elder
	Alder
	Birch
	Oak
	Walnut
	Pine
		Quack grass/
		Wheatgrass
		Redtop
		Vernal grass
		Brome
		Orchard grass
			Pigweed
			Saltbush/Scale
			Lamb's Quarter
			Mexican Firebush
			Russian Thistle
			Ragweed, False,
			  Giant, Short
			  & Western

XVII
CA (North-
western)
WA (Western)
OR (Western)
	Box Elder
	Alder
	Birch
	Hazelnut
	Oak
	Walnut
	Ash
		Bent grass
		Vernal grass
		Oats
		Brome
		Bermuda grass
		Orchard grass
		Salt grass
			Pigweed
			Saltbush/Scale
			Lamb's Quarter
			Russian Thistle
			Ragweed, False,
			  Giant, Short,
			  & Western

(continued...)

Pollen Map and Guide
for the United States *(continued)*

Map area	Trees[1]	Grasses[2]	Weeds[3]
Alaska	Alder Aspen Birch Cedar Hemlock	Blue grass/ June grass Brome Canary grass Fescue	Bullrush Dock/Sorrel Lamb's Quarter Nettle Plantain
Hawaii	Acacia Beefwood Juniper/ Cedar Cypress	Bermuda grass Corn Finger grass Johnson grass Love grass	Cocklebur Plantain Kochia Pigweed Ragweed, Slender

[1]Pollenating season, ordinarily late winter through spring.
[2]Pollenating season, ordinarily spring through early summer.
[3]Pollenating season, ordinarily summer through early fall.
[4]Only the more common and widespread pollens for each area are listed. This pollen guide to the United States is reproduced with permission of Miles Pharmaceutical Division, West Haven, CT. It is reproduced from *Botanical Regions of the United States and Canada,* 1975.

APPENDIX C

Common Dust, Chemicals, and Fumes That Trigger Upper and Lower Respiratory Symptoms

1. House dust
2. Gasoline/petroleum products
3. Household cleaning products
4. Insect repellents
5. Soaps, shampoos, and bath oils
6. Incense
7. Gas fumes
8. Shoe polish
9. Moth balls
10. Formaldehyde
11. Insect bodies
12. Nail polish
13. Cigaret smoke
14. Fertilizers
15. Air spray
16. Photography solutions
17. Plastics

APPENDIX D

Allergens and Irritants Encountered at Home, Work, or in School Triggering Lower Respiratory Symptoms

A. Allergens
  1. House dust
  2. Animal dander
  3. Tree pollen
  4. Grass pollen
  5. Weed pollen
  6. Mold

B. Chemicals
  1. Ozone
  2. Sulfur dioxide
  3. Automobile emissions
  4. Tobacco smoke
  5. Also see Appendix C

C. Infections
  1. Viral infections, especially RSV and influenza
  2. Some bacterial infections

D. Exercise
  1. Especially outdoor running

E. Nonsteroidal anti-inflammatory drugs
  1. Aspirin
  2. Ibuprofen or Motrin
  3. Other drugs commonly used to treat arthritis

APPENDIX E

**Foods Known to Provoke
Allergic or Hypersensitive Reactions[1]**

  1. Milk
  2. Eggs
  3. Soy beans
  4. Peanuts
  5. Fish
  6. Wheat
  7. Celery
  8. Tomato
  9. Shrimp (and other crustacea)

[1]These are the most commonly incriminated foods. However, as noted in the text, there are multiple other problems with foods and, in theory, any food can become an irritant or an allergen.

APPENDIX F

An Elimination Diet

All fruits and vegetables, except lettuce, must be cooked or canned

Foods allowed:

Rice	Pears	Lamb
Rice wafers	Beets	Carrots
Puffed rice	Chard	Lettuce
Rice flakes	Oyster plant	Sweet potato
Rice Krispies	Apricots	Acetic acid vinegar (white)
Cranberries	Peaches	Olive oil, Crisco, or Spry
Salt	Tapioca	Sugar, cane or beet
Water	Vanilla extract, synthetic	

Any vegetable oil except oleo margarine

Eat and drink only the foods listed! Here is a *Suggested Menu*:

Breakfast	*Lunch*	*Dinner*
Rice Krispies	Lamb chop	Lamb patty
Rice wafers	Sweet potato	Boiled rice
Peaches	Beets	Carrots
Apricot juice	Rice wafers	Lettuce with acetic acid
Peach jam	Cranberry juice	Peaches
Water	Pears	Apricot juice

AVOID: Coffee, tea, cola, soft drinks, chewing gum, all medications except those ordered by a doctor.

INSTRUCTION:

- Stay on basic diet for 14 days. If there are no changes in symptoms, then stop the diet. If the diet seems to work, i.e., if the symptoms disappear...
- Then, on day 15 add yellow vegetables all by themselves.
- Then, on day 22 add green vegetables all by themselves.
- Next, on day 31 add chicken all by itself.

Continue adding food groups one at a time at 7-day intervals.
Keep a Diet Diary as indicated. Add foods in large amounts, and eat them several times a day during the addition period.

Appendix G

Food Groupings

1. Apple—apple, pear, quince
2. Aster—lettuce, chicory, endive, escarole, artichoke, dandelion, sunflower seeds
3. Beet—beet, spinach, chard
4. Blueberry—blueberry, huckleberry, cranberry
5. Cashew—cashew, pistacchio, mango
6. Chocolate—chocolate (cocoa) and cola
7. Citrus—orange, lemon, grapefruit, lime, tangerine, kumquat, citron
8. Fungus—mushroom, yeast
9. Ginger—ginger, cardamom, turmeric
10. Gooseberry—currant, gooseberry
11. Grain (cereal or grass)—wheat, corn, rice, oats, barley, rye. Also wild rice, cane, millet, sorghum, bamboo shoots
12. Laurel—avocado, cinnamon, bay leaves, sassafras
13. Mallow—cottonseed and okra
14. Melon (gourd)—watermelon, cucumber, cantaloupe, pumpkin, squash, and other melons
15. Mint—mint, peppermint, spearmint, thyme, sage, basil, savory, rosemary, catnip
16. Mustard—mustard, turnip, radish, horseradish, watercress, cabbage, kraut, chinese cabbage, broccoli, cauliflower, Brussels sprouts, collards, kale, kohlrabi, rutabaga
17. Myrtle—allspice, guava, clove pimento
18. Onion—onion, garlic, asparagus, chives, leeks, sarsparilla
19. Buckwheat—buckwheat, rhubarb, garden sorrel
20. Palm—coconut, date
21. Parsley—carrot, parsnip, celery, celeriac, anise, dill, fennel, angelica, celery seed, cumin, coriander, caraway
22. Pea (legume or clover)—peanuts, peas (green, field, blackeyed), beans (navy, lima, pinto, string, soy), licorice, acacia, tragacanth
23. Plum—plum, cherry, peach, apricot, nectarine, almond
24. Potato—potato, tomato, egg plant, green pepper, red pepper, chili pepper, paprika, cayenne
25. Rose—strawberry, raspberry, blackberry, dewberry, loganberry, youngberry, boysenberry
26. Walnut—black or English walnut, pecan, hickory nut, butternut.

APPENDIX H
Mold-Free Diet

Eliminate:

1. All cheeses including cottage cheese, sour cream, sour milk and buttermilk
2. Beer and wine
3. Cider and homemade root beer
4. Mushrooms
5. Soy sauce
6. Canned tomatoes, unless homemade
7. Pickled and smoked meats and fish, including sausages, hot dogs, corned beef, pastrami, and pickled tongue
8. Vinegar and vinegar-containing foods such as mayonnaise, pickles, pickled vegetables, green olives, and sauerkraut
9. Soured breads (e.g., pumpernickel), fresh rolls, coffee cakes, and other foods made with large amounts of yeast
10. All dried and candied fruits including raisins, apricots, dates, prunes, and figs
11. Melons, especially cantaloupe

APPENDIX I
Tyramine-Free Diet

Eliminate:

1. Chocolate, cocoa, fava beans
2. All ripened cheeses
3. Avocados
4. Bananas
5. Canned figs
6. Yeast extracts
7. Fermented sausage (*i.e.,* bologna, salami, pepperoni, aged beef, hot dogs)
8. Beer
9. Chicken livers
10. Pickled herring
11. Anchovies
12. Dried fish
13. Red wine, sherry

APPENDIX J

Foods Allowed for Cereal-Free Elimination Diet

Tapioca	Carrots	Cane or beet sugar
White potato	Chard	Salt
Sweet potato or yam	Lettuce	Sesame oil
Soy bean potato bread	Lima beans	Soy bean oil
Lima bean potato bread	Peas/Spinach	Willow Run oleomargarine
Soy bean milk	Squash	Gelatin (Knox's), flavored
Lamb	String beans	with allowed fruits and
Beef	Tomato	juices
Chicken, fryers, roasters	Apricots*	Baking soda
Capon	Grapefruit*	Maple syrup or
Bacon	Lemon	syrup made with
Liver (lamb)	Peaches*	cane sugar flavored
Cream of tartar	Pineapple*	with maple
Artichoke	Prunes*	White vinegar
Asparagus	Pears*	Vanilla extract
Beets	Lemon extract	Corn-free baking powder

*The canned fruits should be preserved with cane sugar, not corn sugar.
Water-packed fruits may be used and sweetened with cane sugar syrup.

APPENDIX K

Milk-Free Diet

Eliminate:

1. Milk, including low fat, skim, buttermilk
2. Dairy products
   a. Butter
   b. Ice cream and sherbet
   c. All cheeses
   d. Yogurt
   e. Cottage cheese
   f. Sour cream
3. Common foods that contain dairy products
   a. Puddings

   b. Custards
   c. Cream soups
   d. Breads
   e. Pastry
   f. Spaghetti
4. All foods that contain (read labels)
   a. Non-fat dry milk solids
   b. Sodium (Na) caseinate
   c. Whey
5. Chocolate, cocoa

APPENDIX L

Environmental Protection Agency Offices

Region 1

Environmental Protection Agency
John F. Kennedy Federal Building
Room 2203
Boston, MA 02203
DDD: 617-585-3420

Region 2

Environmental Protection Agency
Jacob K. Javits Federal Building
26 Federal Plaza
New York, NY 10278
DDD: 212-264-2657

Region 3

Environmental Protection Agency
841 Chestnut Building
Philadelphia, PA 19107
DDD: 215-597-9800

Region 4

Environmental Protection Agency
345 Courtland Street, NE
Atlanta, GA 30365
DDD: 404-347-4727

Region 5

Environmental Protection Agency
230 South Dearborn Street
Chicago, IL 60604
DDD: 312-353-2000

Region 6

Environmental Protection Agency
First Interstate Bank Tower
    at Fountain Place
Suite 1200, 12th Floor
1445 Ross Avenue
Dallas, TX 75202-2733
DDD: 214-655-6444

Region 7

Environmental Protection Agency
726 Minnesota Avenue
Kansas City, KS 66101
DDD: 913-551-7000

Region 8

Environmental Protection Agency
999 18th Street, Suite 500
Denver, CO 80202-2405
DDD: 303-293-1603

Region 9

Environmental Protection Agency
75 Hawthorne Street
San Francisco, CA 94105
DDD: 415-744-1305

Region 10

Environmental Protection Agency
1200 Sixth Avenue
Seattle, WA 98101
DDD: 206-442-1200

Appendix M

Addresses and Telephone Numbers of Regional and Area OSHA Offices

Boston—*Region I:* Connecticut, Maine, Massachusetts, New Hampshire, Rhode Island, and Vermont

> *Boston Regional Office*
> US Department of Labor—OSHA
> 133 Portland Street, 1st floor
> Boston, Massachusetts 02114
> 617-565-7164

Boston North Area Office

US Department of Labor—OSHA
Valley Office Park
13 Branch Street, 1st Floor
Methuen, Massachusetts 01844
617-565-8110

Boston South Area Office

US Department of Labor—OSHA
639 Granite Street, 4th Floor
Braintree, Massachusetts 02184
617-565-6924

Concord Office

US Department of Labor—OSHA
Federal Building, Rm. 334
55 Pleasant Street
Concord, New Hampshire 03301
603-225-1629

Providence Office

US Department of Labor—OSHA
Federal Office Building
380 Westminster Mall, Rm. 243
Providence, Rhode Island 02903
401-528-4669

Springfield Area Office

US Department of Labor—OSHA
1145 Main Street, Rm. 108
Springfield, Massachusetts 01103
413-785-0123

Augusta Area Office

US Department of Labor—OSHA
40 Western Avenue, Rm. 121
Augusta, Maine 04330
207-622-8417

Hartford Office

US Department of Labor—OSHA
Federal Office Building
450 Main Street, Rm. 508
Hartford, Connecticut 06103
203-240-3152

New York City—*Region 2:*   New Jersey, New York, and
Puerto Rico

New York Regional Office
US Department of Labor—OSHA
201 Varick Street, Rm. 670
New York, New York 10014
212-337-2378

Manhattan Area Office

US Department of Labor—OSHA
90 Church Street, Rm. 1405
New York, New York 10007
212-264-9840

Long Island Area Office

US Department of Labor—OSHA
990 Westbury Road
Westbury, New York 11590
516-334-3344

Queens Area Office

US Department of Labor—OSHA
42-40 Bell Boulevard, 5th Floor
Bayside, New York 11361
718-279-9060/9050

Albany Area Office

US Department of Labor—OSHA
Leo W. O'Brien Federal Building, Rm. 132
Clinton Avenue and North Pearl Street
Albany, New York 12207
518-472-6085

Syracuse Area Office

US Department of Labor—OSHA
100 South Clinton St., Rm. 1267
Syracuse, New York 13260
315-423-5188

Buffalo Area Office

US Department of Labor—OSHA
5360 Genesee Street
Bowmansville, New York 14026
716-684-3891/4018

Puerto Rico Area Office

US Department of Labor—OSHA
US Courthouse and FOB
Carlos Chardon Avenue, Rm. 555
Hato Rey, Puerto Rico 00918
809-753-4457/4072

Philadelphia—*Region 3:*   Delaware, District of Columbia,
Maryland, Pennsylvania, Virginia,
and West Virginia

Philadelphia Regional Office
US Department of Labor—OSHA
Gateway Building, Suite 2100
3535 Market Street
Philadelphia, Pennsylvania 19104
215-596-1201

Philadelphia Area Office

US Department of Labor—OSHA
US Custom House, Rm. 242
Second and Chestnut Street
Philadelphia, Pennsylvania 19106
215-597-4955

Wilmington District Office

US Department of Labor—OSHA
Federal Office Building, Rm. 3007
844 King Street
Wilmington, Delaware 19801
302-573-6115

Pittsburgh Area Office

US Department of Labor—OSHA
Federal Building, Rm. 2336
1000 Liberty Avenue
Pittsburgh, Pennsylvania 15222
412-644-2903

Erie District Office

US Department of Labor—OSHA
Rathrock Building, Rm. 408
121 West 10th Street
Erie, Pennsylvania 16501
812-453-4351

Wilkes-Barre Area Office

US Department of Labor—OSHA
Penn Place, Rm. 2005
20 North Pennsylvania Avenue
Wilkes-Barre, PA 18701
717-826-6538

Allentown District Office

US Department of Labor—OSHA
850 N. 5th Street
Allentown, Pennsylvania 18102
215-776-4220

Charleston Area Office

US Department of Labor—OSHA
550 Eagan Street, Rm. 206
Charleston, West Virginia 25301
304-347-5937

Atlanta—*Region 4:* Alabama, Florida, Georgia, Kentucky, Mississippi, North Carolina, South Carolina, and Tennessee

Atlanta Regional Office

US Department of Labor—OSHA
1375 Peachtree Street, NE, Suite 587
Atlanta, Georgia 30367
404-347-3573

Atlanta Area Office

US Department of Labor—OSHA
Building 7, Suite
LaVista Perimeter Office Park
Tucker, Georgia 30084
404-331-4767

Savannah Distrtict Office

US Department of Labor—OSHA
1600 Drayton Street
Savannah, Georgia 31401
912-944-4393

Birmingham Area Office

US Department of Labor—OSHA
Todd Mall
2047 Canyon Road
Birmingham, Alabama 35216
205-731-1534

Columbia Area Office

US Department of Labor —OSHA
1835 Assembly Street, Rm. 1468
Columbia, South Carolina 29201
803-765-5904

Jackson Area Office

US Department of Labor—OSHA
Federal Building, Suite 1445
100 West Capitol Street
Jackson, Mississippi 39269
601-965-4606

Mobile District Office

US Department of Labor—OSHA
951 Government Street, Suite 502
Mobile, Alabama 36604
205-690-2131

Chicago—*Region 5:* Indiana, Illinois, Michigan, Minnesota, Ohio, and Wisconsin

Chicago Regional Office

US Department of Labor—OSHA
32nd Floor, Rm. 3244
230 South Dearborn Street
Chicago, Illinois 60604
312-353-2220

Calumet City Area Office

US Department of Labor—OSHA
1600 167th Street, Suite 12
Calumet City, Illinois 60409
312-891-3800

Chicago North Area Office

US Department of Labor—OSHA
2360 E. Devon Avenue, Suite
Des Plaines, Illinois 60018
312-803-4800

Aurora Area Office

US Department of Labor—OSHA
344 Smoke Tree Business Park
North Aurora, Illinois 60542
312-896-8700

Cincinnati Area Office

US Department of Labor—OSHA
Federal Office Building, Rm. 4028
550 Main Street
Cincinnati, Ohio 45202
513-684-3784

Cleveland Area Office

US Department of Labor—OSHA
Federal Office Building, Rm. 899
1240 East 9th Street
Cleveland, Ohio 44199
216-522-3818

Columbus Area Office

US Department of Labor—OSHA
Federal Office Building, Rm. 620
200 North High Street
Columbus, Ohio 43215
614-469-5582

Indianapolis Area Office

US Department of Labor—OSHA
46 East Ohio Street, Rm. 423
Indianapolis, Indiana 46204
317-269-7290

Dallas—*Region 6:* Arkansas, Louisiana, New Mexico, Oklahoma, and Texas

Dallas Regional Office

US Department of Labor—OSHA
525 Griffin Street, Rm. 602
Dallas, Texas 75202
214-767-4731

Dallas Area Office

US Department of Labor—OSHA
1425 West Pioneer Drive
Irving, Texas 75061
214-259-6683

Austin Area Office

US Department of Labor—OSHA
611 East 6th Street, Rm. 303
Austin, Texas 78701
512-482-5783

Albuquerque Area Office

US Department of Labor—OSHA
320 Central Avenue, SW, Suite 13
Albuquerque, New Mexico 87102
505-776-3411

Baton Rouge Area Office

US Department of Labor—OSHA
Hoover Annex, Suite 200
2156 Wooddale Boulevard
Baton Rouge, Louisiana 70806
504-389-0474

Corpus Christi Area Office

US Department of Labor—OSHA
Government Plaza, Rm. 300
400 Mann Street
Corpus Christi, Texas 78401
512-888-3257

Lubbock Area Office

US Department of Labor—OSHA
Federal Building, Rm. 421
1205 Texas Avenue
Lubbock, Texas 79401
806-743-7681

Kansas City—*Region 7:* Iowa, Kansas, Missouri, and
Nebraska

Kansas City Regional Office

US Department of Labor—OSHA
911 Walnut Street, Rm. 406
Kansas City, Missouri 64106
816-426-5861

Kansas City Area Office

US Department of Labor—OSHA
911 Walnut Street, Rm. 2202
Kansas City, Missouri 64106
816-426-2756

St. Louis Area Office

US Department of Labor—OSHA
Washington Avenue, Rm. 420
St. Louis, Missouri 63101
314-425-4249

Des Moines Area Office

US Department of Labor—OSHA
210 Walnut Street, Rm. 815
Des Moines, Iowa 50309
515-284-4794

Wichita Area Office

US Department of Labor—OSHA
216 North Waco, Suite B
Wichita, Kansas 67202
316-269-6644

Omaha Area Office

US Department of Labor—OSHA
Overland-Wolf Building, Rm. 100
6910 Pacific Street
Omaha, Nebraska 68106
402-221-3182

Colorado—*Region 8:*   Denver, North and South Dakota, Utah, and Montana

Colorado Regional Office

US Department of Labor—OSHA
1961 Stout Street, Rm. 1576
Denver, CO 80204
303-844-3061

Colorado Area Office	*Utah Area Office*
US Department of Labor—OSHA	US Department of Labor—OSHA
1244 Speer Blvd., Suite 360	1781 S. 300 West
Denver, CO 80204	Salt Lake City, UT 84115
303-844-5285	801-524-5080

North and South Dakota Area Offices	*Montana Area Office*
US Department of Labor—OSHA	US Department of Labor—OSHA
Federal Building, Rm. 348	19 North 25th Street
Bismark, ND 58501	Billings, MT 59101
701-250-4521	406-657-6649

San Francisco—*Region 9:*   American Samoa, Arizona, California, Guam, Hawaii, Nevada, Trust Territory of the Pacific Islands

San Francisco Regional Office

US Department of Labor—OSHA
71 Stevenson Street, Room 415
San Francisco, California 94105
415-744-7107

Long Beach Area Office	*Walnut Creek Area Office*
US Department of Labor—OSHA	US Department of Labor—OSHA
400 Oceangate, Suite 530	801 Ygnacio Valley Road, Suite 205
Long Beach, California 90802	Walnut Creek, CA 94596/3823
213-514-6387	415-943-1973

Sacramento Area Office	*West Covina Area Office*
US Department of Labor—OSHA	US Department of Labor—OSHA
2422 Arden Way, Suite A-1	100 N. Citrus Street, Suite 240
Sacramento, California 95825	Coast Savings Building
916-646-9220	West Covina, California 91791
	818-915-1558

San Diego Area Office

US Department of Labor—OSHA
5675 Ruffin Road, Suite 330
San Diego, California 92123
619-569-9071

Los Angeles Area Office

US Department of Labor—OSHA
3325 Wilshire Blvd., Suite 601
Los Angeles, California 90010
213-252-7829

Seattle—*Region 10:* Alaska, Idaho, Oregon, and Washington

Seattle Regional Office

US Department of Labor—OSHA
1111 Third Avenue, Suite 715
Seattle, Washington 98101-3212
206-442-5930

Anchorage Area Office

US Department of Labor—OSHA
Federal Building
701 C Street, Box 29
Anchorage, Alaska 99513
907-271-5152

Boise Area Office

US Department of Labor—OSHA
Room 324, Federal Building/USCH
550 West Fort Street, Box 007
Boise, Idaho 83724
208-334-1867

Bellevue Area Office

US Department of Labor—OSHA
121-107th Street, NE
Bellevue, Washington 98004
206-442-7520

Portland Area Office

US Department of Labor—OSHA
1220 Southwest 3rd Ave., Rm. 640
Portland, Oregon 97204
503-221-2251

APPENDIX N

Medic-Alert Procedure

If you are subject to severe or life-threatening reactions to allergens or irritants, you should take two precautions:

1. Carry appropriate treatment medications with you at all times, and know how and when to use them. For acute allergic or hypersensitive episodes this emergency resource will ordinarily be an ANA-Kit or Epi-Pen, which your doctor must prescribe for you. The kit contains antihistamines and a syringe pre-loaded with epinephrine.

2. Secure and wear Medic-Alert identification (bracelet or necklace) which will register your problem at Medic-Alert's central registry and will signal and specify your problem to anyone called on to provide you with emergency treatment. Medic-Alert applications can be secured from your physician, your HMO, or by writing to:

> The Medic-Alert Foundation
> PO Box 1009
> Turlock, CA 95381-1009

APPENDIX O

Detection and Strategies for Managing Radon

Several chapters of this book contain sections dealing with radon, an invisible, odorless, tasteless, radioactive, carcinogenic gas resulting from the decay of uranium. It is found in soils and rocks containing uranium, granite, shale, phosphate, and pitchblende, and in soils holding certain industrial wastes.

The presence of radon can be detected by using either a charcoal canister or an Alpha Track Detector. Information about obtaining these test kits and how to use them can be secured from your state radiation protection service or office, usually a unit of the State Health Department. The test kits cost anywhere from $25 to $50.

Once obtained and used, the test kits must be sent away for laboratory analysis. The results will be reported to you and will give you information on interpreting them and suggesting additional steps you may need to take.

You may find it helpful to contact the Environmental Protection Agency (EPA) office nearest to you for advice and help. EPA addresses are given in Appendix L. The EPA has issued a helpful booklet entitled *A Citizen's Guide to Radon: What It Is And What To Do About It,* which may be purchased from the Superintendent of Documents, US Government Printing Office, Washington, DC, 20402.

APPENDIX P

Air Cleaning and Filtering Sources

Chapter 12 identifies the various types of air conditioning or air purifying devices in use, describes and appraises the various filters employed in them, and offers suggestions to follow in finding, selecting, installing, and using the unit most practicable for you. It also notes that *Consumer Reports* periodically tests and rates air cleaners, and the Association of Home Appliance Manufacturers maintains a list of certified room air cleaners. The table below summarizes information on room-sized units using various kinds of filters.

Type of filter	Purchase price	Monthly rental	Filter costs	Remarks
Electronic/ electrostatic	$300 and up	$40 and up	N/A	Filter must be washed regularly; some noise; some models generate high levels of the irritant, ozone
HEPA (high efficiency particulate arresting)	$400 and up	$50 and up	$40– 80	Replace filter screen every 18 months; some noise; over 5 years will cost 50% more than comparably priced electrostatic unit
Fiber	$100 and up	$15 and up	$5– 20	Replace filter screen monthly; some noise; less efficient than HEPA; some models ineffective
Ionizing	Up to	Up to	N/A	Charged particles go to clean surfaces; quiet; units and capacities small, more than one needed for large room; some models ineffective

Appendix Q

Sources of Information About and Suppliers of Allergen and Irritant-Managing Products

The best starting points for information about and names of suppliers of irritant or allergen-managing products are the Yellow Pages of your telephone directory or the Allergy Products Directory, which is available from the Allergy Publications Group, PO Box 640, Menlo Park, CA 94026-0640 at a cost of $9.95.

Here are some of the Yellow Page headings you may find helpful in locating local suppliers of needed materials or supplies:

Air Cleaning and Purifying Equipment
Air Conditioners
Air Conditioning Equipment and Systems—Repairing
Clean Room—Installation and Equipment
Dust and Fume Collecting Systems
Dust Control Materials
Environmental and Ecological Services
Health Appliances
Health and Diet Food Products—Retail
Hospital Equipment and Supplies
Safety Equipment
Water Filtration and Purification Equipment
Water Softening and Conditioning Equipment—Service and Supplies

The Health and Well-Being, Home Interior and Decorating, and House Remodeling and Garden indexes of the "smart" Yellow Pages will also provide leads. In addition, ask your physician, HMO, or allergist to suggest local sources of supply.

We have listed below some of the more frequently-sought devices or materials needed by individuals with allergies or hypersensitivities, and the names of a few of their suppliers. However, these mentions should not be taken as an endorsement of any firm, product, or service named.

We have observed that enterprises specializing in allergic products or services tend to have short life expectancies; therefore, we have made no attempt to compile a comprehensive listing of resources, knowing that it would be outdated soon after publication.

General Suppliers

Large mercantile chains (Montgomery Ward, J.C. Penney, Sears, etc.) carry some of the products that people affected by allergens or irritants may require. Some others include:

Allergy Control Products
96 Danbury Road
Ridgefield, CT 05877
203-438-9580

The Allergy Store
PO Box 2555
Sebastopol, CA 95473
800-824-7163

The AL-R-G Shop
3411 Johnson St.
Hollywood, FL 33021
305-981-9182

Bio-Tech Systems
PO Box 25380
Chicago, IL 60625
800-621-5545

Environmental Corporation
PO Box 31313
St. Louis, MO 63131
800-423-1982

Cotton Bedding/Apparel

Some soft goods retailers—Eddie Bauer, L.L. Bean, Orvis, etc.—offer untreated cotton products as part of their merchandise lines.

The Company Store
500 Company Store Road
LaCrosse, WI 54601
800-323- 8000

The Cotton Place
PO Box 59721
Dallas, TX 75229
800-451-8866

Dona Designs
825 Northlake Dr.
Richardson, TX 75080
214-235-0485

Garnet Hill
262 Main
Franconia, NH 03580
800-622-6216

Janice Corporation
198 Route 46
Budd Lake NJ 07828
800- JANICES

Vermont Country Store
Weston, VT 05161
802- 824-6932

Food and Food Products

There is an impressive number of small and essentially local businesses that sell various allergy or irritant-related products. Some of these suppliers are listed in the *Allergy Products Directory* that we referred to earlier in this Appendix; others will be found in your locality by turning to the Food Products or Health and Diet Food Products—Retail listings in the Yellow Pages. As we note in Chapters 6 and 10, special caution needs to be exercised in using and accepting the claims put forward for foods or food additives touted to be safe or helpful for individuals with food allergies or hypersensitivities.

The American Academy of Allergy and Immunology has published a *Grocers Manufacturers of America Contact List* that provides names of contact persons who can supply information on ingredients of manufactured foods. Your allergist will have or know how to secure and use this resource.

Masks / Respirators

A.J. Masuen Company
PO Box 768
Elk Grove Village, IL 60009
800-831-0894

Mine Safety Appliance Co.
519 Niagara St.
Tonawanda, NY 14150
716-691-6922

Nebulizers

De Vilbiss Health Care Worldwide
PO Box 635
Somerset, PA 15501
814-443-4881

DURA Pharmaceuticals Inc.
PO Box 28331
San Diego, CA 92128
619-789-6840

Paints, Finishes, Sealers, Household Cleansers, etc.

Non-allergic or non-irritant alternatives or strategies are available for most of these common chemicals. Chapter 11 identifies some of them. In addition, there are free publications available that will tell you how to avoid using (or how safely to use) caustics, corrosives, solvents, paints, aerosols, pesticides, herbicides, automotive products, and medications. Check with your local Toxic Information Center or Poison Control Center for information. Baubiologie Hardware, 207 Sixteenth St., Unit B, Pacific Grove, CA 93950, 408-372-8626 has a catalog that features many of these alternative products.

Vacuum Cleaners (House Dust and Mite Specific)

Nilfisk of America Inc.
300 Technology Drive
Malvern, PA 19355
800-NILFISK

Sanyo
21350 Lassen Street
Chatsworth, CA 91311-2329
818-998-7322

Index